Good Nutrition for a Healthy Menopause

Good Nutrition for a Healthy Menopause

Louise Lambert-Lagacé

Translated by Fred Reed and Charles Phillips

Published in 1999 by Stoddart Publishing Co. Limited
34 Lesmill Road, Toronto, Canada M3B 2T6

Original French edition published in Quebec
in 1998 by Les Éditions de l'Homme

Distributed by:
General Distribution Services Ltd.
325 Humber College Blvd., Toronto, Canada M9W 7C3
Tel. (416) 213-1919   Fax (416) 213-1917
Email customer.service@ccmailgw.genpub.com

03 02 01 00 99   1 2 3 4 5

Canadian Cataloguing in Publication Data

Lambert-Lagacé, Louise, 1941-
Good nutrition for a healthy menopause

Translation of: Ménopause, nutrition et santé.
Includes bibliographical references and index.
ISBN 0-7737-6073-3

1. Menopause – Nutritional aspects. 2. Middle aged women – Nutrition.
3. Middle aged women – Health and hygiene.
I. Reed, Fred A., 1939–   . II. Phillips, Charles. III. Title.

RG186.L3513 1999   618.1'750654   C99-931463-7

Cover Design: Angel Guerra
Text Design: Tannice Goddard

THE CANADA COUNCIL | LE CONSEIL DES ARTS
FOR THE ARTS | DU CANADA
SINCE 1957 | DEPUIS 1957

*We acknowledge for their financial support of our publishing
program the Canada Council, the Ontario Arts Council, and
the Government of Canada through the Book Publishing
Industry Development Program (BPIDP).*

Printed and bound in Canada

Contents

Acknowledgements

There's a story behind every book. This book's story is a particularly happy one. Without the tender loving care and encouragement of the many friends who shaped a sheltering, positive environment for me, it surely would not have become what it is today: a reliable source of information for women reaching menopause.

Jacques Laurin, publisher of Les Éditions de l'homme, got me off to a running start when he accepted my proposal. I owe him my deepest gratitude not only for saying "yes" but for helping me, in his inimitable way, to maintain my initial impetus. Lise Guertin, his right-hand woman, gave invaluable assistance through her constructive comments on the first draft of my manuscript.

Roxane Duhamel, my associate in the Québec Business Women's Network, kept me company throughout the actual writing process, by reading and responding to each chapter. No author could hope for a finer first reader.

Jérémie Thériault and Marilène Gagné, interns in dietary science, did the hard bibliographical slogging. They did the real footwork, too, tracking down hard data on the supermarket shelves. Jérémie brought his remarkable critical faculties to bear on several key chapters. Their contribution is highly appreciated.

Last but not least, my young colleague, dietitian Caroline Dubeau, worked overtime to sift through the raw information and shape it into a harmonious whole. Without her contribution, this book — my eleventh — would not be what it is today.

Several women, young and not so young, read the manuscript and shared their comments and criticisms with me. My thanks to Noella Lacasse, Lise Garneau, Christiane Desjarlais and my daughter Pascale for their time and their encouragement.

Health-care professionals were also generous with their knowledge and skills. I confess however that what I feared most were their criticisms! Warmest thanks to Diane Corbeil and Andrée Chatel — your positive remarks lent me wings. Thanks as well to my two close associates Louise Desaulniers and Michelle Laflamme.

At Stoddart, once more Nelson Doucet believed in me and my topic. Fred Reed and Charles Phillips were successful in translating the book's text as well as its tone, which is so precious to an author. Marnie Kramarich and her team edited the book with patience and good humour. It made my work so much easier. Many thanks to you all.

It remains only for me to wish a long and active life to the English-language translation of *Good Nutrition for a Healthy Menopause*.

Why I Wrote This Book

*T*his is a book on nutrition written specifically for that period in a woman's life known as the menopause. Writing it has been a pleasure. I feel as though I'm pursuing an ongoing dialogue. In my previous book *The Nutrition Challenge for Women*, my goal was to convince you of the importance of proper nutrition all through your life. My aim was to help you develop a more harmonious relationship with the food you eat, and of course to encourage you to eat healthier foods. In *Good Nutrition for a Healthy Menopause*, I concentrate on several specific menopause-related disorders and suggest diet-based solutions to deal with them. I also take up longer-term issues such as preventing osteoporosis and cardiovascular disease, and introduce you to several can't-miss food combinations.

I was 42 years old when I first took an interest in the menopause — not mine but other women's. It was then that I planned and chaired a series of workshops on menopause organized by the University of

Montreal public lecture program, Les Belles Soirées de l'Université de Montréal. I knew next to nothing about the subject. I had to learn almost everything from scratch. But I felt certain that one day all of the information I'd accumulated would prove useful. Sixteen years and some 30 workshops later, I've gained a much better grasp of my material — and my subject. I owe much to my fellow conference chair-women, one of them a physician, Diane Corbeil, and two psychologists, Nicole Trudel and Andrée Chatel, who shared with me not only their immense storehouse of knowledge, but also their own thinking about this crucial mid-point in every woman's life.

When we presented our first workshops back in 1983, research on the importance of diet in menopause barely existed. How the field has changed since then! For example, researchers in Europe and the United States have looked much more closely at weight gain during menopause. Many others have measured the effect of different types of fat on the female arteries, where previously they had been almost exclusively concerned with those of the male. Researchers in Finland and Australia have identified the presence of hormones (the phytoestrogens) in certain foods and confirmed their effect on the hot flashes associated with menopause. Others evaluated the quantities of calcium and other nutritive elements needed to preserve bone health and to combat osteo-porosis. The antioxidants found in foods and dietary supplements were also subjected to exhaustive scrutiny. This growing body of research made it possible for me to develop a much more sophisticated nutritional approach than ever before, and to draw up a diet that's a winner from start to finish.

I first applied this knowledge in my own nutrition clinic and in my own life. Today, I am convinced that the impact of certain menopause-related disorders can be lessened by eating the right food at the right time. I've come to believe that menopause provides an exceptional opportunity to change the way we live our lives, to pay closer attention to our health and, in the process, to prepare ourselves for healthy aging. The certainty that a healthful, well-planned diet can make a difference, that such a diet is within reach of all women, but that it was not sufficiently well known, gave me the stimulus to write this book.

In it, I provide new nutritional information to give you relief from hot flashes, to help you find new energy, to reduce bloating, control weight and reduce the risk of cardiovascular illness, osteoporosis and breast cancer. By combining this information with what you already know, you will draw fuller enjoyment from this new stage in your life. I have not taken up some of the wider questions associated with menopause, problems such as irritability, memory loss, shifting sleep patterns and changes in sexuality. All are fascinating topics, but fall outside the scope of this book.

I argue neither for nor against hormone replacement therapy. In this book, the accent is on a dietary approach adapted to the menopause. I consider it a complement to treatment with hormones, in the event you have opted for that approach.

For me, menopause is as normal as it is natural. It happens to every woman. It is not an illness, nor a deficiency-related problem.

After a close and detailed study of the latest medical literature, I now have a better understanding of the action and impact of hormone replacement therapy. I admit that, for a wide variety of reasons, some women may need or wish to use hormones. Many women who take hormones on a regular basis attend my nutrition clinic; some are in top shape. I have also encountered women who began taking hormones, experienced adverse reactions and were obliged to stop. Still others are in splendid form, but are neither able nor willing to take hormones in any way, shape or form. I now view hormone replacement therapy as a personal choice and, in certain cases, as a question of health.

But I do react sharply when I read about or hear the kinds of promises being made to women concerning the benefits of hormone replacement therapy. The information that is given is rarely accurate or complete. Research into the benefits of hormones continues, and not all the answers are in yet, as outstanding researchers in the field are prepared to admit.

I would never deny that there are as many kinds of menopauses as there are women of menopausal age. No two women pass through this stage of life in exactly the same way. However, I do know that each and every one of us must eat three meals a day. A diet better adapted to our needs and physical vulnerabilities can only be beneficial.

My own menopause was uneventful. I come from a healthy family background. I chose not to take hormones for the simplest of reasons: I wanted to grow old on my own terms, relying on my own means.

Of course, menopause is also a time for talking about prevention. Prevention of cardiovascular disease, osteoporosis and breast cancer. Each, I admit, is an important consideration. But prevention is not the main reason I look after my health and urge you to look after yours. It's a question of caution, of wisdom, but above all, it's a question of love.

For me, health is a treasure that I do not take for granted. It is so precious that once lost it cannot be restored easily. I give it all the tender, loving care I can; I safeguard it jealously to draw the maximum benefit for the longest possible time.

I know that healthy living habits, a diet adapted to my lifestyle, and regular physical activity are the tools to do the job. What motivates me is not the fear of illness. No — it's the powerful impulse to enjoy what life has to offer for many years to come. Experiencing menopause in a positive way and growing old in good health means taking care of what I enjoy being.

I've written my book in this spirit — a spirit I hope you will find in the pages that follow.

I

Growing Old,
Staying Healthy

*I*t's hard not to notice menopause. It affects our bodies, our minds, our hearts and the image we see in the mirror. But menopause is also a normal part of every woman's life, a hormonal transition phase that affects our entire being. Why shouldn't every woman use it as a unique opportunity to rethink her lifestyle and diet? To redefine what she wants to become? One thing is certain: every woman wants to maintain her good health for as long as she possibly can.

Menopause may amount to little more than another stage in the long process of growing old, but when it does arrive, it forces us to look at aging more seriously than we did when we were 30. Sometimes I find myself wondering if growing old is permitted in a society ruled by the cult of youth. I look around me and I see women struggling valiantly against the tell-tale signs of growing old, against folds of flesh, sagging skin, white hair and wrinkles, courtesy of a protective and preventive arsenal that did not even exist a short few years ago. While I respect their choice, I cannot help but admire the women who swim against the current, who decide to grow old as naturally as they can.

"When people look at a woman, they don't see her wrinkles, they see her charm. Women really have to be more generous with themselves and with others; they have to learn to like themselves," responded a remarkably vivacious actress in her sixties when asked about aesthetic surgery.

Today, with the image of the svelte young woman ever present, it may be the perfect time to redefine the beauty of maturity and advancing age, and help ourselves step with serenity into the sixth and seventh decades of our lives.

"A woman who has reached maturity, a woman who is at the height of her powers, who looks upon the world and her fellow human beings with wide-open eyes and a touch of irony, a woman who has been touched by life, tested, often betrayed but who has not lost her faith in herself . . . how much more fascinating, more admirable she is than a young woman without a history," I read one day — and have never forgotten it.

When I gave my first workshops on menopause a good 16 years ago, I found myself surrounded by elegant, eye-catching women with a youthful, dynamic look about them but who were experiencing real difficulties related to menopause. Their handsome appearance surprised me; I had a slightly different perception of menopausal women. Since then, I've brought my ideas into line with reality, with good reason. . . .

A woman at menopause is still young, even if she's begun to grow a little older. But who doesn't grow old?

"Youth is not a period of one's life. It's a state of mind, an effort of will, a quality of the imagination, an emotional intensity . . .

"We only grow old when we abandon our ideals."

Douglas MacArthur (1880–1964)

AGING ISN'T WHAT IT USED TO BE

In years gone by, the process of growing old sprinkled life with a fine dust that would build up over the years, gradually isolating the aging woman from the society around her. Old age was to be suffered passively and in silence. Today, even people of 75 or older are no longer resigned, isolated senior citizens. Many maintain busy schedules and contribute to the well-being and betterment of the society around them. Many travel, ski, garden, play golf or swim. They do everything they can to keep in excellent physical condition and take an active interest in their own well-being. These people are the new models for the golden-age years.

The April 1998 issue of the *New England Journal of Medicine* profiles the findings of a study of 1,700 individuals who were recruited in their forties and were monitored for 36 years. The authors of the article concluded that non-smokers, those who maintained a normal weight and who kept up regular exercise lived longer and in better health than those with less healthy habits.

Instead of searching for eternal youth and beauty, preserving a quality lifestyle over the long run is what gives me my motivation. It is the principal objective of my nutritional approach to menopause.

MENOPAUSE: MYTH AND REALITY

Only recently has menopause emerged from the dark closet of taboo and into the light of public discussion, friendly chit-chat, curiosity and even humour. It may bring with it the usual catalogue of discomforts, but it rarely leaves any lasting ill effects. Quite the contrary, in fact. A California study involving 600 women between the ages of 50 and 89 showed that 55% of those surveyed said life had gotten better after menopause, 57% were happier than they had been before, despite the hot flashes, weight gain, night sweats, fatigue, insomnia and irritability they experienced. A mere one woman in 10 admitted that she did not enjoy growing older.

Another survey, carried out in the summer of 1997 by the North American Menopause Society among 750 women ranging in age from 45 to 60, revealed that a majority of women considered menopause as the point of departure for a new, fuller life. Only 11% of those surveyed saw it as a negative experience.

Menopause may well be one of those life passages that aren't necessarily easy to negotiate. But compared to adolescence, it's smooth sailing!

In fact, many women are surprised to find that they've grown stronger in emotional, spiritual and physical terms. They've acquired a sense of plenitude, of confidence in their capacity for life. Some of them eliminate the superfluous things and make a new beginning, enriched by the period of hormonal turbulence they've passed through. As the French philosopher Michel Serres writes: "Interesting things happen in times of turmoil."

Menopause can be a time for taking stock of your ideas, your feelings. Use it to make changes in your routine, in your daily life, in your work and in your leisure-time activity. And you've got the perfect excuse! You're learning to grow old in good health.

I was almost impatient to begin my own menopause. I wanted to compare what I would experience with all the things I had read and heard. When it came, I took the opportunity to make significant changes in the way I lived. I found time to do more than just work. Before the age of 45 I hadn't been involved in any physical activity. Since then, I have learned to put my muscles and bones to the test and gained confidence in the strength of my own body. Now I ski, play tennis and hike — with the greatest of pleasure. I make every effort to savour life's precious moments, for the loss of friends of the same age set me to thinking about the end point of our voyage on this earth.

Today, I'm proud to have two grandsons and a granddaughter. I never imagined I would experience such intense feelings of love!

A NEW DIETARY APPROACH

A healthy, varied diet has long been recognized as one of the most useful tools for preserving good health. A diet adapted to the specific needs of menopause can provide us with yet another tool. It may not be as well known, but it is a tool of great promise. The latest research tends to indicate that certain foods can ease the discomfort associated with menopause, and that other foods can lessen the risk of illness over the longer term. We cannot afford to ignore the findings of the most recent dietary research.

No doubt you are aware of the link between calcium and bone health, but you may not have realized how much more complex the story really is. Rather than considering calcium as the sole indispensable element, current research places a much greater accent on the complementary nutritive elements that can either increase or reduce bone density.

You may have heard of the hormones present in certain foods, such as soy products. In this book, you will discover the numerous advantages of regular consumption of the hormones known as phyto-estrogens, the scientific name for estrogen derived from plants.

Have you already tried unsuccessfully to lose weight? The information in the following pages will help you gain a deeper understanding of what happens at menopause, and of what you should eat to stay healthy.

Do you sometimes feel you left your energy in the closet at your thirtieth birthday? You can rediscover it by adopting a winning dietary routine.

You will make the acquaintance of boron and other substances that either stimulate, or interfere with, hormonal circulation.

Are you absolutely sure that you have chosen the foods that lower bad cholesterol (LDL) while raising good cholesterol (HDL) levels as a way of lowering the risk of cardiovascular disease?

Do you carefully select which antioxidants you consume, either in your food or in the form of supplements, to slow the aging process?

By improving the nutritional component of your menu, you will find the energy you thought you'd lost, reduce your hot flashes, protect your bones and blood vessels and keep your weight under control.

Paying more attention to the food on your plate means making the most of your menopause, and growing old in good health.

Where do we stand today?

Today, more and more research is being focused on premenopausal and post-menopausal women. Most such studies have focused on hormonal replacement therapy. Very little research has evaluated the nutritional aspect.

We hear through the grapevine that women are often poorly nourished at the onset of menopause.

- The obsession with slimness persists, along with its perverse side effects. In fact, the situation may be getting worse. What are we to think of the women who have used fashionable appetite-reducing drugs such as fenfluramine or dexfenfluramine? Thirty percent of them now suffer from a rare cardiac valve malformation. Though their case is not quite as serious, what of the women who have followed all the weight-loss diets on the market without ever having reached a healthy weight, or worse, having put more weight back on?
- Not necessarily related to the above, many women simply put on weight with age, even though they eat less and less.
- Even though fat consumption has been dropping over the last several years, hydrogenated fat consumption remains excessive. A daily intake of more than two grams of this type of fat increases the risk of cardiovascular disease in women by more than 21% (see Table 1, page 8). Heavy consumption of saturated fats (meat and cheese) adds another element of risk.
- From adolescence on, women do not consume adequate quantities of foods rich in calcium. In fact, instead of increasing with age as recommended by experts, calcium consumption is dropping. The intake

of vitamin D and other minerals is likewise deficient; as a result, bone health suffers.

- For many women, the usual protein intake throughout the day is clearly inadequate. The near-absence of protein at the morning and midday meals explains the sudden onset of tiredness at the end of the morning and at four o'clock in the afternoon. It is also explains the sugar cravings that so many women experience.
- Consumption of foods rich in zinc, magnesium, vitamin B6 and folic acid has not reached satisfactory levels, which may well have an adverse effect on the nervous and cardiovascular systems.
- The lack of dietary fibre remains acute and may well explain why constipation and diverticulitis are more frequent after menopause.
- The consumption of fruits and vegetables rich in potassium and magnesium is too low to prevent or alleviate the problems of hypertension that often appear after age 50.

These dietary deficiencies may not be tragic, but they certainly don't help women experience a discomfort-free menopause. On the contrary, they can cause and worsen such serious problems as hypoglycemia, diabetes, insulin resistance, reduced thyroid activity, increased bad cholesterol (LDL) and decreased good cholesterol (HDL).

> If you really want to ease your passage through menopause and grow older in good health, you need to modify your eating habits. Your efforts will be rewarded. It's never too late to make the right decision!

TABLE 1
Foods Rich in Trans Fatty Acids*

Food	Portion	Trans fat (g)
Potato chips	1 small bag	7.0 – 9.0
Corn chips	1 small bag	5.7 – 6.5
Hydrogenated margarine	15 mL (1 tbs.)	3.0 – 6.0
Doughnut	1	2.8 – 3.3
Shortening	15 mL (1 tbs.)	2.2 – 2.6
French fries	small portion	1.3 – 1.7
Muffin (fast food)	1	1.1 – 1.7
Cake	1 slice	1.0 – 3.0
Chocolate	1 bar	0.9
Pizza crust	small	0.6 – 0.8
Cookies	1	0.3 – 2.0
Crackers	1	0.4 – 1.0
Some dry cereals	1 bowl	0.2 – 0.7

* Trans fatty acids are found in hydrogenated fats.

II

Our Changing Waistlines

Whether it's in Italy or Mexico, Toronto or Montreal, when menopause arrives, nearly all the women in the world put on some weight. But whatever we call our extra kilos — mid-life fullness, or new curves in old places — they are rarely welcome.

Rather than shed tears, protest or even stop eating, wouldn't it be better and wiser to understand the changes taking place inside our bodies, and to manage their impact on us?

Remember, you're not alone. A survey done by a Quebec women's magazine showed that nearly 75% of 465 women respondents (aged 50 to 65) put on weight — between 5.5 and 6.8 kg (12 and 15 lb.) — over the course of their menopause. Population studies in both Canada and the United States during the last 50 years bear out the gradual increase in women's weight between ages 25 and 60, with the sharpest increase usually taking place between 45 and 55.

OUR CHANGING BODIES

As women grow older, their bodies change both internally and externally, even if their weight remains relatively stable. For example, a woman of 60 whose weight has not changed throughout her adult life no longer has the same muscle or bone structure that she had at age 30. The same weight may show on the bathroom scale, which is itself unusual, but the composition of her body is no longer the same, which is entirely normal.

Let me illustrate what I mean. An elegant businesswoman in her early sixties confided to me last fall that she had not put on an ounce since age 20. But, she added, her waistline had expanded from 56 to 70 cm (22 to 27 in.), and her shape was no longer the same.

As a rule, a woman entering her forties experiences a loss of muscle tissue of about 0.5 kg (1 lb.) every three years. For the period covering the pre-menopause to the post-menopause, the loss is higher, about 3 kg (6 1/2 lb.).

Roughly the same rule applies to our bones. We experience a yearly loss of 1% from age 30 onward, and from 2% to 5% per year during menopause itself. During the sixth and seventh decades, the pace of loss slows, fluctuating between 0.5% and 1% per year (see Chapter 7).

A FEW MORE HOLES IN THE BELT

In our fifties, excess weight is no longer located in the same spots, and no longer has the same impact on health.

When you were younger and put on weight, the excess fat settled in your hips and thighs. This fat was relatively inert and hard to lose, but it presented few long-term side effects.

But women who gain weight during menopause tend to accumulate adipose tissue around the waist and in the lower abdomen. This new fat tissue is metabolically more active. It is located closer to the liver and the pancreas, increases the danger of diabetes and may touch off an increase of bad cholesterol and triglycerides.

Certainly, a few extra kilos have very little effect, especially if your weight remains within your healthy weight zone (see Table 2, page 24). This healthy weight zone corresponds to a Body Mass Index (BMI) of between 20 and 25, which is associated with a low risk of illness.

> If you are 1.6 m (5′3″) tall and weighed 55 kg (120 lb.) at age 35, your BMI was 21. At 50, you weigh 61 kg (135 lb.) and your BMI is 24. As both BMIs, 21 and 24, fall within the healthy weight zone, you run no greater risk of illness.

A BMI of more than 26 starts putting your health in jeopardy. The more fat that accumulates around the waist, the greater the risk of developing diabetes or cardiovascular disease. After an exhaustive study of the question from all possible angles, a health research team led by Laval University's Dr. Claude Bouchard concluded that the risk of illness increases when a woman's waist measure exceeds 85 cm (33 in.). His findings suggest that, in order to minimize risk, a woman should keep her waistline below 75 cm (29 in.) during menopause.

I've added two or three kilograms (4 1/2 to 6 1/2 lb.) over the last five years. These extra kilos have settled directly behind the last button on my blazer. I've become an expert in letting out waistbands that have become too tight and offsetting the buttons on my jackets. Nowadays I look for clothing that lets my waist breathe, and I tend to buy slightly larger sizes. An ounce of prevention is worth an hour of unstitching!

EXTRA FOOD OR EXTRA STRESS?

There is no single simple explanation for weight gain at menopause. Contrary to what one might think, women eat less and less as they grow older, a fact confirmed by all nutrition surveys. Other research indicates that there is not necessarily a correlation between the quantity of fat consumed and a thickening at the waistline. The notorious mid-life weight gain cannot be explained by abusive food intake; in fact, the opposite is true. Several researchers have pointed to stress as the factor that may accelerate the deposit of intra-abdominal fat. Indeed, the changes that many women experience in their lives at menopause may well increase stress.

A SLOWER METABOLIC RATE

The fall-off in the body's own production of estrogen that takes place at menopause causes the metabolic rate — the rate at which a certain number of calories are burned every day — to slacken. This shift happens gradually from age 30 onward, but accelerates as estrogen levels begin to fall. The fewer calories your metabolism can burn in 24 hours, the more likely you are to gain weight.

Physical activity not only offsets the slowing of your metabolic rate. It also builds up muscle mass that burns more calories than fatty tissue. Unfortunately, too many women are unaware of this fact. No sooner do they reach their fiftieth birthday than they hang up their skates and consign their skis and tennis rackets to the closet. When they do so they actually contribute, without realizing it, to lowering their body's calorie-burning capacity.

Worse yet, too many women skip meals without considering how it might affect their metabolism. They end up actually harming themselves, for the metabolism always interprets the absence of food for more than a few hours as a period of starvation. It reacts the only way it can: by slowing down calorie combustion. The damage becomes particularly visible during the years that precede the complete cessation of menstruation.

Weight loss diets also have a direct effect on the metabolic function: the stricter the diet, the more drastic the slowdown. The greater the frequency of dieting, the less efficient your metabolism. Some women who have followed such diets while neglecting exercise will gain weight from eating practically nothing when they reach menopause.

Metabolism is a poorly understood function: it manages the transformation of calories into energy by burning a certain number of calories every 24 hours in order to maintain all the functions of the human body.

When it receives fewer calories to burn, or when you skip a meal, it shifts into energy-saving mode, maintaining the same body functions with less fuel. Our body adapts so well that it can survive famine or a low-calorie diet. On the other hand, it strongly resists long-term weight loss, which it interprets as a threat to survival.

After a low-calorie diet, the metabolism has difficulty recovering its former combustion capacity. It continues to burn calories at a slower rate and favours the build-up of fat stores in anticipation of the next period of famine or the next diet.

This explains the notorious weight-gain rebound in the months or years that follow a diet.

A CHANGE OF LIFE?

Other changes in our bodies that have nothing to do with hormones may take place at menopause and explain a weight gain. For instance, a new partner with a big appetite can turn your eating habits upside down. A new job that demands less physical effort, or early retirement that slows down your daily routine, can have an impact on the energy you expend. Chronic back pain or sore feet may keep you from exercising. Perhaps you've stopped smoking and put on from 4.5 to 6.6 kg (10 to 15 lb.) without eating a bite more than before. As you can see, even simple changes in your life may explain an increase in weight.

A BEAUTY BONUS, A HEALTH BONUS

The extra weight that comes at menopause is neither harmful nor useless. Look at the women around you who are growing old gracefully. They look healthy, their faces are full and they have glowing cheeks and smooth skin. Now look at the impact of weight loss on a 60-year-old woman. You will surely agree that a thin face ages less well than a full face. We could even say that at menopause, a loss of weight creates the impression of sudden aging, while a weight increase makes women look younger.

On the good-health side, the fat stored at menopause promotes the transformation of another sex hormone: androstenedione. This hormone, produced by the adrenal glands, is transformed into estrogen in the fatty tissues and plays the role of a back-up hormone, circulating throughout the body and relieving certain disorders. After menopause, the more fatty tissue in the body, the greater the quantity of back-up estrogen in circulation. This added dose of fat and estrogen strengthens the bone structure and explains why plump women have fewer fractures than thin women.

At Toulouse University hospital, in France, a group of 50 women of normal weight at least five years beyond menopause were tracked for 40 months. Researchers who measured the bone density of the women noted a significant link between weight gain and bone mass retention; the women who had gained more than 1 kg (2 1/4 lb.) had less than half the bone loss of the women who had gained no weight.

Now we understand why osteoporosis specialists like to see women fill out a bit. They know that higher weight provides greater protection against fractures, while subnormal weight increases the risk of osteoporosis.

A study by the National Institute on Aging carried out on 3,700 women and published in 1996 noted a significantly increased risk of hip fracture among women who lost 5 to 10% of their body weight after age 50. The research team observed that a woman of 50 with a healthy height-to-weight ratio who lost 10% of her weight doubled her risk of hip fracture. For example, a woman of 55 who weighs 59 kg (130 lb.) and with a Body Mass Index of 22 (healthy weight) doubled her risk of fractures if she lost 5.8 kg (13 lb.) or more. When she loses weight, she loses both muscle and fat tissue; she has less estrogen in circulation, and a smaller protective cushion of fat around her hips. Obviously, a plump woman who loses a few kilos hardly runs the same risk as a thinner one.

Gerontologists have also focused on the impact of weight gain and loss over the course of an adult life. One of them, Dr. R. Andres of the United States National Institute of Health, reviewed 13 major studies on longevity among different population groups. Contrary to what one might think, he concluded that people who gain weight during their adult life generally live longer than those who maintain the same weight or lose weight.

Gaining weight is not compulsory, but of course maintaining a healthy weight offers better protection. Still, slimming at all costs is not recommended, especially if your weight already falls within the healthy weight zone.

Women who remain slim after menopause are more vulnerable to fractures, but they remain less susceptible to diabetes, cardiovascular disease and breast cancer, none of which is to be taken lightly. What's more, they have no need to change their wardrobe.

You may be a little full-figured, or a little slim — but you can still grow old in good health.

THE EFFECT OF HORMONES

The debate may be never-ending, but recent research indicates that there is no significant difference in weight gain between women who take hormones and those who do not.

Dr. John F. Aloia's team at Winthrop University Hospital in Mineola, New York, followed 118 women from ages 50 to 55 for a period of three years. The women were divided into three segments: a control group; a second group, which took calcium supplements; and a third group, which used a combination of calcium supplements and hormone replacement therapy. At yearly intervals the research team measured the women's fat tissue, muscle mass and bone density. At the end of the three years there was a greater weight gain among the women who had received hormone therapy, but all the women had put on some fat and lost a little muscle.

At the Jerusalem University Hospital menopause clinic, Dr. Benjamin E. Reubinoff's team investigated the impact of hormone replacement therapy on the weight of women who had just begun menopause. The survey covered 63 women ranging in age from 44 to 54 who were monitored for a year. Half of them received hormone replacement therapy; the other half acted as a control group. All the women gained from 1.5 to 2 kg (3 1/4 to 4 1/2 lb.).

Another study carried out in Italy examined the weight, fat distribution and hormonal balance of 600 women between 45 and 65. The researchers observed that post-menopausal women weighed significantly more than their pre-menopausal counterparts. Weight increase was progressive; no difference was observed between women who received hormone replacement therapy and those who did not.

The famous PEPI (Post-menopausal Estrogen/Progestin Interventions) study, copiously cited in the scientific literature, monitored 875 women divided into five groups over a three-year period. The first group received no hormones, while the other four did, but in varying dosages. The study concluded that:

- Half the women, whether taking or not taking hormones, gained less than 2.5 kg (5 1/2 lb.).
- Nineteen percent of women taking hormones and 18% of women not taking hormones gained between 2.5 and 4.9 kg (5 1/2 and 11 lb.).
- Smokers who took hormones gained 1 kg (2 1/4 lb.) more than smokers who did not.
- Women who were very active physically but did not take hormones lost 0.7 kg (1 1/2 lb.), but equally active women who did take hormones gained 0.9 kg (2 lb.).

Several women who attend my clinic complain of increased weight after taking hormones; some even stop taking them in order to lose a few kilos. Before going to such extremes, let's look at ways of recovering a more balanced approach to the food we eat.

PATHWAYS TO A SOLUTION

Women have had their fill of weight-loss diets. They're fed up with fasting and calorie counting.

The other day, a woman walked into my clinic with a sad story. She'd spoiled 30 years of her life attempting to lose weight. She is not the only woman to have lived through such a trying experience. Today she refuses to count calories and to go to bed ravenous with hunger, but she wants to find a well-balanced menu.

I was delighted with her attitude. The suggestions found in this book are bound to please her and women like her. They all point to another way of eating, better suited to this period of rapid hormonal change.

1. Adopt an anti-diet approach.

If you've put on a bit of weight over the last few years, you should be aware that the years preceding and following the end of menstruation are the least favourable for weight loss. Many studies have confirmed the fact. At one time you could lose weight with a little effort; now you simply cannot. Your body has reorganized itself to deal with the hormonal transition and now it seems to resist every attempt to lose weight. What should you do?

- If your weight still falls within the healthy weight zone (see Table 2, page 24), you're better off carrying a few extra kilos and staying in good shape rather than risking a nutritional deficiency and triggering sudden aging.
- If your weight has been well beyond the upper limits of the healthy weight zone for several years, don't rush into another diet. Rethink your strategy. Instead of fasting with no real weight loss, try to slow

down the weight gain. Your body will respond better a few years down the line.

The anti-diet approach I suggest doesn't mean eating whatever strikes your fancy in whatever quantity. It's simply a way of encouraging you to forget calorie counting and the bathroom scale.

Fill your plate with foods rich in minerals, fibres and vitamins — the substances that will see you through a carefree menopause. You'll be pleasantly surprised.

A 1996 Italian study of breast cancer risk factors demonstrated that it is possible to lose weight without counting calories. The research team recruited 100 women between the ages of 50 and 65. Half of them were asked to regularly eat soy, flaxseed, nuts, leafy green and cruciferous vegetables, small fruits, whole cereal products and fish. They were also asked to reduce their consumption of meat, cheese, sweets and refined foods, but were given no restrictions as to amounts. The remaining 50 women acted as a control group and made no changes in their food intake.

Six months later, the first 50 women — those who had eaten all the extra vegetables, fruits, whole grains, nuts and soy they wished — had lost 3.8 cm (1 1/2 in.) around the waist and more than 4 kg (8 3/4 lb.), as well as lowering their cholesterol levels, their blood sugar and their cancer risk. Those women who did not change their diet did not lose weight, nor were their other risk factors reduced.

Their case is only one of many. I could multiply the examples by the number of women I see in my nutrition clinic, women who have obtained similar results just by improving their food choices.

2. Avoid the no-fat trap.

You've become a bit of a fanatic when it comes to choosing your food: fat-free salad dressings, low-fat cheese and ice cream, no-fat cookies . . . Well, you're not alone. It's a typical American trend that's become contagious and jumped the border. Unfortunately, it just doesn't do what it's cracked up to do: Americans eat 11% less fat than they did 20 years ago, their calorie intake is down by 4%, they consume tons of diet foods — and the incidence of obesity has soared by 31% since 1976, according to a report published in the *American Journal of Medicine* in 1997. I guess you could call it "the American paradox."

You can escape this trap by choosing good fats like olive or canola oil for your salad dressings, or by eating nuts for a snack; go easy on fried foods and items rich in hydrogenated fats (see Table 1, page 8). Your menu will be much more nutritious and your weight will not soar.

3. Increase your vegetable intake.

If you are like most women in Canada, you probably eat fewer vegetables than you should. Perhaps you manage two servings a day, but that's not enough.

An epidemiological study of some 80,000 individuals between ages 40 and 54 carried out in the United States over a 10-year period set out to isolate the cause of overall mid-life weight gain. The researchers took into account the habits of the study participants, including their marital status, education, and use of vitamin supplements, tobacco and alcohol. They concluded that those who gained less weight were those who consumed more vegetables, ate less meat and exercised regularly. Their vegetable intake exceeded 20 servings per week, which is by no means an enormous quantity, but does indicate a healthier-than-average diet.

In my clinic, women who manage to eat from four to six portions of vegetables per day are more successful than others in losing weight. The extra vegetables replace other, richer foods and provide a wide range of potentially beneficial nutritive elements.

If you prefer fruit, consuming them in abundance will certainly help you — but as a complement, not a replacement for your vegetables.

If you hardly know where to begin, chose any one of these easy suggestions:

- Try a new vegetable or fruit every week.
- Double your usual portions of vegetables.
- Add fruit to your cereal: a banana, a sliced apple, green or red grapes, strawberries or blueberries, tangerines — the choice is yours.
- Prepare sparkling juices by combining carbonated spring water with fruit juice.
- Prepare little bags of raw vegetables to nibble on as is or with dips while you cook.
- Add vegetables to your favourite spaghetti sauce: mushrooms, green or red bell peppers, cauliflower or broccoli, or grated carrots.
- Cook up tasty side dishes with vegetables and/or fruits, apple, endive and nut salad; carrot salads with raisins; spinach salad with tangerine segments; zucchini-stuffed tomatoes with herbs, avocado and grapefruit salad, or ratatouille.
- Prepare one hearty soup per week using vegetables in season: leeks, mushrooms, asparagus, tomatoes, green peas, spinach; make extra quantities and freeze, then warm up in the microwave when you get that famished feeling.
- Be bold; try the less well-known greens like arugula, Swiss chard and Napa cabbage — you'll boost your intake of vitamins and minerals.

4. Eat smaller meals.

You may not have realized it, but it's healthier to eat several smaller meals in the course of a day than one large one, especially as you grow older. A recent study showed that while young women can easily burn off a meal of 1,000 calories, older women don't have the same capacity. When they eat large meals, they simply store the fat they haven't been able to burn and put on weight.

Fat combustion takes place first and foremost in the muscle tissue and provides the fuel for exercise. When physical activity and muscle mass diminish, as they do at menopause, women lose their capacity to burn large quantities of fat at the same meal. Remember: for women 40 and over, small meals burn better than big ones.

5. Never skip a meal.

I often encounter women in their fifties who cannot explain their weight gain because they eat little more than an evening meal. They skip breakfast because they're not hungry, skip lunch due to lack of time, and end up ravenous at suppertime. So they rush through their evening meal and snack away until bedtime. And they gain steadily. When these women adopt a three-meals-a-day routine, they're pleasantly surprised. At last, they succeed in losing some weight.

When you go without food for several hours, you send a starvation message to your metabolism, which in turn slows down combustion and switches into saving mode. When you begin eating regularly again, you re-set your metabolism to normal. It may take a while, but it will happen.

The secret lies in adopting a three-meals-a-day routine. If you're hungry and you foresee a few extra hours before your next meal, have a snack. If not, the hunger message will kick in. Remember that skipping meals leads you directly to cravings, and cravings never help!

6. Increase your physical activity.

Regular physical activity is vital to maintaining weight — and health. As people turn 50, they become less and less active. The Canadian Institute for Research on Physical Condition reports that in Quebec, 63% of the population is inactive. Even if you have cut back your calorie intake, your weight will continue to increase if you do not exercise regularly. Why? Because without physical activity, the metabolism slows right down and is unable to offset the drop-off in calorie combustion that usually accompanies weight loss diets and menopause itself. But if you become more active, you can develop your muscle mass and increase your capacity to burn fat. You can even eat a little more without putting on weight. You may even lose a few centimetres from your waist.

Not quite convinced? A Colorado-based research team measured the metabolic rate of 65 healthy women with stable body weights. The group included younger and older women, some of them sedentary, others quite active. Among the inactive, they noted that menopausal women had a metabolic rate that was 10% slower than that of the younger women. But among the more active, they detected no difference between the metabolic rate of the younger and older subjects. It follows that a more rapid metabolic rate accompanies a greater muscle mass and a smaller weight gain.

Physical activity can also prevent a weight regain in the months or years that follow a significant weight loss. Janice Thompson's research team at the University of North Carolina measured the impact of physical activity on menopausal women who wanted to lose weight. She monitored three groups of women, two of which only reduced their calorie intake, while the third group added three hours of walking and two hours of weight resistance training to their weekly routine. After six months, the women in all three groups had lost weight but the third group now had a more rapid metabolic rate. Meanwhile, women in the third group who continued with their program of physical activity after the completion of the study lost from one to two additional kilograms (2 1/4 to 4 1/2 lb.) while the sedentary subjects quickly put back 1 1/2 kg (3 1/4 lb.).

Still other researchers have concluded that, to maintain a new, healthier weight after a weight loss diet and to keep up the metabolic rate, it is necessary to engage in 80 minutes of moderate exercise, or 35 minutes of more intense exercise, every day.

7. *Reduce your alcohol and tobacco consumption if necessary.*
Extra weight stored at the waist increases the risk of diabetes and the accumulation of bad cholesterol; the greater the excess weight, the greater the danger. Researchers from Dr. Claude Bouchard's Laval University team looked long and hard at the question. They identified alcohol and smoking as two harmful factors that have a greater impact on fat deposits than fat consumed from the diet. Other studies have shown that smokers who took hormone replacement therapy gained on average 1.1 kg (2 1/2 lb.) more than those who took no hormones.

One thing is certain: alcohol and nicotine will not improve any woman's health as she grows older.

> Don't forget that it's easier to lose a few pounds a few years after the complete cessation of menses than during the pre-menopausal period.

TABLE 2

Body Mass Index (BMI) — Shaded area is "Healthy Weight Zone"

Weight

Height (ft.)	(m.)	46 (100)	48 (105)	50 (110)	52 (115)	55 (120)	57 (125)	59 (130)	61 (135)	64 (140)	66 (145)	68 (150)	71 (155)	73 (160)	75 (165)	77 (170)	80 (175)
		(kilos) (lbs)															
4'9"	1.45	22	23	24	25	26	27	28	29	30	31	33	34	35	36	37	38
4'10"	1.47	21	22	23	24	25	26	27	28	29	31	32	33	34	35	36	37
4'11"	1.50	20	21	22	23	24	25	26	27	28	29	30	31	32	33	34	36
5'	1.52	20	21	22	23	24	25	26	27	28	28	30	31	32	33	33	35
5'1"	1.55	19	20	21	22	23	24	25	26	27	27	28	29	30	31	32	33
5'2"	1.58	18	19	20	21	22	23	24	25	26	27	28	28	29	30	31	32
5'3"	1.60	18	19	20	21	21	22	23	24	25	26	27	28	29	29	30	31
5'4"	1.63	18	18	19	20	21	21	22	23	24	25	26	27	27	28	29	30
5'5"	1.65		18	18	19	20	21	22	22	23	24	25	26	26	28	28	29
5'6"	1.68		17	18	19	19	20	21	22	23	24	24	25	26	27	27	28
5'7"	1.70		17	17	18	19	20	20	21	22	23	24	24	25	26	27	28
5'8"	1.73			17	18	18	19	20	20	21	22	23	24	24	25	26	27
5'9"	1.75				17	18	19	19	20	21	22	22	23	24	25	25	26
5'10"	1.78				17	17	18	18	19	20	21	22	22	23	24	24	25
5'11"	1.80					17	18	18	19	20	20	21	22	22	23	24	25
6'	1.83					16	17	18	18	19	20	20	21	22	22	23	24

CALCULATING THE BODY MASS INDEX

The healthy weight zone is derived from the Body Mass Index (BMI). The formula is calculated as follows: the Body Mass Index (BMI) equals the weight in kilograms divided by the square of the height in metres. Table 2 (opposite) makes the calculation simple:

1. Find your height in the left-hand column.
2. Follow the corresponding line until you find your weight indicated at the top of the table.
3. Circle the figure where the two meet: this is your index.
4. Compare your own index with the following data:

- an index that falls between 20 and 25 corresponds with an optimal healthy weight;
- an index of 26 or 27 falls into the intermediate, or portly, zone;
- an index exceeding 27 falls into the obesity zone and increases the risk of illness;
- an index lower than 20 falls into the thinness zone and also corresponds with an increased risk of illness;
- a woman who measures 1.65 m (5'5") and weighs 50 kg (110 lb.) has an index of 18, falling below the healthy weight threshold;
- a woman who measures 1.55 m (5'1") and weighs 59 kg (130 lb.) has an index of 25, falling into the healthy weight zone;
- a woman who measures 1.68 m (5'6") and weighs 61 kg (135 lb.) has an index of 23, falling into the healthy zone.

III

Yesterday's Energy Today

For many women, menopause means feeling tired day in and day out for no particular reason. Some feel like a shadow of themselves; their energy seems to melt away like snow in the spring sun. Others experience a sudden drop in energy at specific times of the day, as if they've run out of gas. More than a few have told me they just don't feel like their old selves; even making it through the day has become a problem. Still others report shaking or cold sweats.

THE CAUSES OF FATIGUE
The hormonal reorganization that takes place at menopause can have both a direct and an indirect impact on your energy level.

Sleep loss caused by hot flashes and night sweats certainly doesn't make it any easier to feel in top shape.

On the strictly dietary level, the little omissions that might have passed unnoticed at age 30 can leave you feeling totally wrung out today. Fortunately, once they've been properly identified, they can be easily corrected. Here are the most frequent:

Poor protein distribution throughout the day. You may be too rushed to eat a proper breakfast so you gulp down a cup or two of coffee on rising, or a muffin and coffee at the office. But that alert, energetic feeling barely lasts a couple of hours. You end your morning feeling worn-out and half-starved. It's time to realize that a serious lack of protein to start off the day can affect your well-being not only before noon, but for the better part of the afternoon as well.

Perhaps you're one of those busy people who always seem to forget to eat a midday meal: there's just not enough time to get everything done. So you replace a full meal with an apple and a pot of yogurt between two phone calls. Once again you risk running out of steam at around four o'clock, with a craving for sugar in the bargain. Not enough protein at lunchtime is the main reason for your problem.

You sincerely believe that a midday meal can consist of a mix of greens in a hearty salad, or a plate of raw veggies. Perhaps it would be a better idea to call it a snack with high vitamin content if the vegetables are carefully chosen, but it's certainly not the kind of square meal that can keep you going throughout the day. Once again, proteins are almost absent.

Come evening, with a ravenous appetite, you wolf down a huge portion of poultry, meat or fish. Then you take a piece of cheese, a bowl of yogurt or a glass of milk with a few cookies. Now you're overdoing the protein — eating too much at one meal.

Eating this way does not stabilize your energy. Instead, it increases your fatigue. To maintain a higher level of energy from morning to night, learn to include protein-rich foods in every meal, and don't skip meals (see Pathways to a Solution, page 31).

Your body absolutely demands the right fuel at the right time in order to perform its job properly. When the right fuel is not a part of your menu, you quickly begin to notice signs of distress. At menopause, these signs will be even more apparent.

Starch, starch and more starch. With the best of intentions, you have cut back on meat in an effort to reduce your saturated fat intake. An excellent decision — but not always the best solution. So you end up with a plate of pasta for lunch. It's the kind of meal, rich in starch, that satisfies your appetite for a while, but won't keep you going for long. Why? Because that plate of pasta stimulates a significant secretion of insulin that triggers intense tiredness later in the afternoon; it can also leave you with the appetite of a lumberjack long before dinnertime.

You're not the only one who likes pasta. A food that turns up so often on restaurant menus can be difficult to avoid.

Not too long ago I found myself in a Montreal department store at the noon hour. Since I'm incapable of skipping a meal, I headed straight for the take-out counter where I beheld perhaps a dozen dishes based on rice, pasta or couscous garnished with vegetables of every size, shape and color. Not a single one of them provided a sufficient quantity of protein. There was only one protein-rich, chicken-based dish, which I immediately ordered.

Even marathon runners are now being told by sports nutrition experts not to overdo their consumption of pasta or other starchy food prior to or during a sporting event. I recently fine-tuned the diet of a 60-year-old female long-distance walker. Before coming to my clinic, she was unable to finish a walk of 50 km (31 miles) because of inadequate protein intake and extensive starch consumption. I drew up a program for her consisting of smaller protein-rich, easy-to-digest meals. Now she can complete a 75-km (47-mile) hike in fine form. A few months ago, she called to tell me about her most recent accomplishment: 100 km (62 miles), using the same menu.

The obsession with slimness. The obsession with slimness does not necessarily disappear with age, and when the menopause adds a couple of centimetres to the waist, it can pop up again. When it does, you find yourself facing a double dilemma: how to eat well and lose weight all at once.

If you attempt to lose weight by regularly skipping meals, your energy will suffer and your weight will not go down — I can guarantee it (see page 21)!

If you peck at your food like a bird, you won't fly too high. Old habits will come back to haunt you. There's even a danger that you won't be able to restrain yourself; you'll end up overeating at your next meal and feeling even more tired once again.

Re-read Pathways to a Solution in Chapter 2, and safeguard your energy.

Iron deficiency. In the years leading up to menopause, menstruation can become more frequent and more abundant. The loss of blood brings with it an additional loss of iron, the principal carrier of oxygen in the blood. When iron and oxygen levels are low, energy declines; breathing becomes laboured and resistance to infection diminishes.

If you normally consume plenty of milk or cheese, you are fulfilling your daily calcium requirement. But your daily food intake may still be short on iron.

If you've systematically replaced red meat with chicken or fish, and if your consumption of soy products or legumes is almost nil, you run the risk of iron deficiency.

If you're not eating plenty of fruits and vegetables at each meal, you are endangering your absorption of iron.

In the past, women needed less iron after age 50. Menopause coincided with the end of menstruation and of blood loss. Today, with hormone replacement therapy, the menopause does not necessarily mean the end of blood loss. If you experience a loss of blood every month, even after menopause, your need for iron remains high, and you should continue to consume adequate quantities of iron-rich foods.

If blood tests show that your hemoglobin levels are barely reaching the normal zone, your iron reserves (ferritin) are probably low. This may be the reason you are always feeling tired. If your hemoglobin level is below normal, you will feel even greater fatigue.

Check this chapter's Pathways to a Solution for the remedy.

Too much heavy food. You succumb to the temptation of fried foods and cream sauces because they're part of the midday special or because they come with the dish.

You drink a glass of wine at lunch to be like everyone else at the table. And if a slice of cake, a piece of pie or a creamy dessert pops up on the special, you eat that too.

These sweets may burn off easily enough after a couple of hours on the ski slopes, a brisk walk or a spin on your bicycle, but if you go straight back to your computer or to your desk, they stick to your ribs. Worse, they make it harder to digest, make your liver and pancreas work harder, and leave you feeling more tired than ever.

Other possible causes of fatigue. If the diet-related pitfalls I've outlined don't really correspond to your situation, your fatigue may have an underlying, organic cause.

- The thyroid gland, which works at processing food into fuel, slows down when estrogen levels fall. A drastic drop can lead to a hypo-thyroid condition, which is more common in women than men after age 40. This type of problem not only undermines your energy but can cause weight gain, cholesterol increase, low tolerance to cold, constipation, dry skin and hair loss.
- Insulin, the hormone that distributes sugar throughout the body, often loses its effectiveness at menopause. It responds less and less well to the demands placed on it, and forces the pancreas to produce more. You become insulin resistant and can have frequent symptoms

related to hypoglycemia. You end up feeling very tired, especially after meals or snacks rich in sugar or starch.

- Diabetes may eventually develop, causing even greater fatigue and imposing substantial changes in your diet. Nearly half of all cases of diabetes appear after age 55, and 60% of these new cases are diagnosed among women.

These illnesses, one of whose symptoms is fatigue, must be diagnosed by your physician, following analysis of blood test results. Thus,

- TSH level measures how well the thyroid gland is functioning;
- fasting insulin level measures insulin resistance;
- induced hyperglycemia measures sugar tolerance;
- fasting blood sugar level indicates whether you are diabetic.

If blood analysis shows an abnormal drop in the thyroid function, you must take the appropriate medication. If fasting insulin and blood sugar levels are abnormally high, you must follow a special, personalized diet to correct the imbalance.

If analysis results are normal and you still feel tired, review your diet while following these recommendations:

Pathways to a Solution
1. Eat the right amount of protein at every meal.
Your body needs the right fuel at the right time. Protein makes up the fuel that can sustain energy for hours on end.

At our nutrition clinic, we make a practice of applying the rule of 15 g of protein per meal, and most of our clients rapidly experience renewed energy (see Table 3, page 35). Whether you are a vegetarian or a meat-eater, you do not need more than 60 g of protein per day, but make sure you take at least 15 g of protein at each and every meal (see Tables 4 and 5, pages 36 to 38).

At breakfast, if you have 250 g (1 cup) of yogurt or 45 g (1 1/2 oz.)

of cheese, or even 250 mL (1 cup) of milk, in addition to a fruit and a cereal product, you've added 10 g of protein to your meal. Try Creamed Tofu with Fruit (recipe on page 47); vary your breakfast menu and obtain the proteins you need to keep you going.

At lunch, add 100 g (3 oz.) of tuna, salmon or chicken to the crispy lettuce and fresh vegetables at the salad bar. You can also add 90 g (1/2 cup) of chick peas or cottage cheese to your vegetable plate.

Dinnertime is a different story. If your serving of poultry, fish or meat is generally copious, don't hesitate to cut back. But do increase your consumption of vegetables. For dessert, take fruit. These few changes won't turn your menu upside down, but they will give you the right amount of protein at the right time, and help you keep your energy up throughout the day.

Consult the menus suggested in Table 5, page 37, and gradually adapt your diet to follow them.

2. Don't hesitate to snack.

We sometimes are under the impression that a healthy diet and between-meal snacks don't mix. In fact, the opposite is true. Snacks can improve the nutritive value of your daily menu and give you the right fuel at the right time.

Some women begin their day between 6 and 7 o'clock in the morning and don't wind down until almost midnight. Others expend large amounts of physical energy or engage in sport-related activities that affect meal times. In such cases, and in so many others, snacks are a must.

No one is suggesting that you eat just anything, anytime — but that you choose foods that can boost your energy for a couple of hours. Protein-rich foods like nuts, yogurt, roasted chick peas or roasted soy beans, a glass of cow's milk or soy milk are excellent examples.

"A little pot of yogurt at 10 o'clock keeps my hunger under control and makes it easier for me to have a normal appetite for my midday meal," a reader wrote me. Choose your snacks from among the foods that provide 5 g or more of protein (see Table 6, page 39).

3. Reduce your sugar intake.

Sugary foods (candies, chocolates, carbonated beverages, even unsweetened fruit juices) and refined foods (white bread, white rice, crackers, cookies, etc.) supply short-term energy only. They temporarily raise blood-sugar levels, stimulate insulin secretion and touch off the sharp drops in energy that we often identify as episodes of hypoglycemia. These foods undermine your energy stability.

If you are one of those women who nibble on sweets as a pick-me-up, forget sugary foods and rely on nutritious snacks instead (again, see Table 6).

4. Limit your alcohol consumption.

The glass of wine that relaxes you can also have the impact of a body blow when you're feeling tired already.

Over the years I've seen many women complain of fatigue. Some of them ate well enough, but would drink one or two glasses of wine every evening. After cutting out wine for a few weeks, they felt much less tired and more alert.

When our body is rested, wine is easy to handle. When it is not, wine can make us even more tired.

5. Eat more iron-rich foods and promote their absorption.

If your iron intake was inadequate before menopause and your blood test results are now at the lower limit of the acceptable range, increase your regular consumption of iron-rich foods.

Here are a few ways you can fortify your menu:

- Incorporate soy in many forms; this legume is high in iron content. You can replace a glass of cow's milk with a soy-based beverage once a day; try tofu-based sauces or spreads.
- Cook a fillet of trout rather than sole or halibut; you'll harvest three times the iron.
- Prepare more iron-rich legume-based dishes.

- Let yourself go a few times a month: try fresh or smoked oysters. They contain more iron than a steak.
- Think again about organ meats such as liver and kidneys; try liver paste or lamb kidneys with *pistou* — all iron-rich delicacies;
- Sweeten your yogurt with a bit of black strap molasses or prune purée, both of them as tasty as they are rich in iron;
- Incorporate into each meal a fruit or vegetable rich in vitamin C, such as oranges, broccoli, bell peppers or cantaloupe to promote iron absorption (see Table 7, page 40).
- Take an iron supplement for three or four months if your hemoglobin or your ferritin levels are low.

> Always look for the right fuel at the right time. Slowly but surely you'll build up your energy.

TABLE 3

Foods that provide 15 g of protein

Food	Quantity
Cooked organ meats: heart, liver, kidneys	90 g (3 oz.)
Cooked seafood: crab, shrimps, lobster, oysters, scallops, etc.	
Cooked game: venison, pheasant, partridge, guinea-hen, etc.	
Cooked fish: halibut, salmon, sole, trout, etc.	
Cooked meat: lamb, beef, pork, veal	
Cooked poultry: turkey and chicken	
Ordinary tofu, firm	90 g (3 oz.)
Ordinary or light ricotta, cottage cheese	135 g (1/2 cup)
Silken tofu, firm	180 g (6 oz.)
Cooked legumes: lentils; red, white, black beans; chick peas, split peas, etc.	180 g (1 cup)
Hard cheeses: Cheddar, Emmenthal, etc.	60 g (2 oz.)

TABLE 4
Some food combinations that provide 15 g of protein*

Combination	Quantity required
Light **ricotta** or **cottage cheese** and **almonds**	90 g (1/3 cup) ricotta or cottage cheese 25 g (3 tbs.) almonds
Small **crab** salad with **cheese** cubes	30 g (1 oz.) crab 45 g (1 1/2 oz.) cheese
Firm silken **tofu**, creamed, with mixed **nuts**	120 g (4 oz.) tofu 25 g (3 tbs.) nuts
Shredded **chicken** and cooked **chick pea** salad	30 g (1 oz.) chicken 90 g (1/2 cup) cooked chick peas
Legume soup with grated **Parmesan cheese**	250 mL (1 cup) soup 12 g (1 tbs.) Parmesan
Yogurt and **walnuts**	175 g (3/4 cup) yogurt 25 g (3 tbs.) walnuts
Black bean and cooked **shrimp** salad	120 g (2/3 cup) cooked black beans 30 g (1 oz.) shrimp
Hard-boiled **egg** salad with cooked **lentils** and **cheese** strips	1 egg 45 g (1/4 cup) cooked lentils 25 g (3/4 oz.) cheese
Beef and **red bean** chili	30 g (1 oz.) beef 90 g (1/2 cup) cooked red kidney beans
Tomato sauce with **lentils** and grated **Parmesan cheese**	125 mL (1/2 cup) sauce 12 g (1 tbs.) Parmesan

* Foods shown in boldface type contain protein.

TABLE 5
Sample menus

Low-protein menus (less than 5 g)	Protein*-rich menus (15 g)
Banana	Banana
Toast	Toast
Strawberry jam	**Peanut butter**
	Glass of **milk**
Orange	Orange
Buttered bagel	Bagel with **ricotta cheese**
Coffee	Coffee with **milk** (café au lait)
Half grapefruit	Half grapefruit
Toasted raisin bread	Toasted raisin bread
	Soft-boiled egg
	Glass of **milk**
Fresh fruit plate	Fresh fruit plate
Crusty roll	**Nuts**
	Vanilla-flavoured **yogurt**
Vegetable soup	Soup made from dried **legumes**
Roll	Roll
Fresh strawberries	**Yogurt** and fresh strawberries
Tomato juice	Tomato juice
Vegetable couscous	Vegetable and **chicken** couscous
Apple	Apple and **almonds**
Rice salad with red pepper	Rice salad with red pepper
Applesauce	**Feta cheese**
Muffin	**Yogurt**

TABLE 5 cont'd
Sample menus

Low-protein menus (less than 5 g)	Protein*-rich menus (15 g)
Raw vegetables	Raw vegetables
Tabbouleh (parsley and cracked wheat salad)	Tabbouleh and **chick peas**
Pear	Pear and **walnuts**
Cucumber spears	Cucumber spears
Tomato sandwich	**Salmon** sandwich
Muffin	Fruit and **sunflower seeds**
Vegetable juice	Vegetable juice
Green salad	**Tuna** and green salad
Oatmeal cookie	Kiwi fruit and **yogurt**
Raw vegetables	Raw vegetables
Spaghetti sauce with vegetables	Spaghetti sauce with **lentils** and grated **Parmesan**
Grapes	Grapes

* Foods shown in boldface type contain protein.

TABLE 6
Foods that provide 5 g of protein

Food	Portion
Almonds or sesame seeds	25 g (3 tbs.)
Almond, sesame or peanut butter	15 mL (1 tbs.)
Soy beverage	125 mL (1/2 cup)
Milk	125 mL (1/2 cup)
Yeast (Torula, Engevita, Red Star)	16 g (2 tbs.)
Walnuts, Brazil nuts, cashews, pistachios, sunflower seeds	35 g (4 tbs.)
Eggs	1
Powdered milk	16 g (2 tbs.)
Powdered soy protein	4 g (1 tsp.)
Spirulina	10 g (2 tsp.)
Tofu spread	45 mL (3 tbs.)
Yogurt, kefir	125 mL (1/2 cup)

TABLE 7
Sources of iron in common foods

Food	Portion		Iron (mg)
FRUITS AND VEGETABLES			
Spinach, cooked	90 g	1/2 cup	3.2
Prune juice	250 mL	1 cup	3.0
Potato, baked	1 medium		2.8
Spirulina	10 g	2 tsp.	2.7
Apricots, dried	8 medium		2.5
Mango	170 g	1 cup	2.1
Figs	5		2.1
Parsley	30 g	1/2 cup	1.9
Green peas, cooked	80 g	1/2 cup	1.2
Brussels sprouts, cooked	80 g	1/2 cup	0.9
Broccoli, cooked	80 g	1/2 cup	0.7
CEREAL PRODUCTS			
Potato flour	90 g	1/2 cup	5.4
Enriched farina, cooked	125 g	1/2 cup	8.0
Shreddies, Raisin Bran	40 g	3/4 cup	5.7
Wheat germ	30 g	1/4 cup	2.1
All Bran	20 g	1/4 cup	1.9
MEAT AND OTHER SOURCES OF PROTEIN			
Tofu, regular	100 g	3.5 oz.	10.5
Atlantic oysters, raw	90 g	3 oz.	6.0
White kidney beans, cooked	180 g	1 cup	5.1
Liver (beef, calf), cooked	90 g	3 oz.	4.9
Chick peas, cooked	180 g	1 cup	4.7
Lima beans, cooked	180 g	1 cup	4.5
Pumpkin seeds, roasted	17 g	2 tbs.	4.1
Black beans, cooked	180 g	1 cup	3.6
Shrimp, cooked	90 g	3 oz.	2.8
Trout, grilled	90 g	3 oz.	2.1
Beef, cooked	90 g	3 oz.	2.0

TABLE 7 cont'd

Sources of iron in common foods

Food	Portion		Iron (mg)
MEAT AND OTHER SOURCES OF PROTEIN CONT'D			
Turkey, lamb, cooked	90 g	3 oz.	1.7
Sesame seeds	20 g	2 tbs.	1.4
Tuna, canned	90 g	3 oz.	1.3
Sunflower seeds, cashew nuts	20 g	2 tbs.	1.0
Chicken, pork, cooked	90 g	3 oz.	0.9
OTHER			
Black strap molasses	15 mL	1 tbs.	3.4

Recommended iron intake for good nutrition:

13 mg/day: menstruating women, women with withdrawal bleeding;

8 mg/day: non-menstruating women (Canada, 1990)

IV

Hot Flashes

*W*hew! If menopause had a trademark, hot flashes would likely be it. They are usually the first, and the most widespread, symptom of the hormonal shift that takes place in every woman's body. But in reality, they are simply evidence of a minor deficiency in our internal thermostat, which no longer seems to know whether we're hot or cold. With little or no warning, women feel a sudden onrush of fever-like heat, particularly in the upper back. It may last for a few seconds, or for several minutes. Red splotches may appear around the throat or on the face, often accompanied by abundant perspiration. When hot flashes occur at night, usually with outbreaks of perspiration — night sweats — they awaken us abruptly and can lead to insomnia.

THE JAPANESE SECRET
More than eight out of 10 North American women complain of hot flashes compared to only two of 10 in Japan, notes McGill University's

Margaret Lock. Professor Lock spent several years in Japan studying menopause in that country first-hand. So unexpected were her conclusions that the international scientific community sat up and took notice.

Not only do Japanese women experience a much lower incidence of hot flashes, they also present four times fewer cases of breast cancer, suffer less from cardiovascular illness and osteoporosis, and live longer than women in the West, she found.

Many researchers have attempted to shine further light on these differences. Some of them have focused on diet. A Finnish research team led by Dr. Herman Adlercreutz was already aware of the presence of estrogenic substances in certain foods. It set out to evaluate how much of these substances normally occurs in the food consumed by Japanese women. The team members measured the quantity of phytoestrogens (see inset) eliminated in the urine of test participants. They detected concentrations from 100 to 1,000 times greater than in the urine of American and Finnish women and were able to establish a direct correlation between excreted phytoestrogens and consumption of tofu, miso, soy and other soybean products (see Table 8, page 51).

> In the mid-80s, scientists confirmed the presence of estrogenic substances in some plant-derived foods. These they named *phytoestrogens*. These substances, inactive in the foods themselves, are transformed into active estrogen by the intestinal flora and have a chemical structure similar to that of the estrogen produced by our ovaries.
>
> They are found principally in soy in the form of isoflavones, and in flaxseed, in the form of lignans.

As you can imagine, more than a few scientists have attempted to examine the effect of phytoestrogens on the symptoms associated with menopause. Research has been under way for some time, and the early results are fascinating.

- Before menopause, the estrogenic activity of the phytoestrogens is weaker than that of estradiol, the estrogen produced by our ovaries. Nonetheless, these phytoestrogens are capable of competing with our own estrogen by using the same receptors. In doing so, they seem to act as antiestrogens that researchers believe may be particularly useful in the prevention of hormonally dependent cancers such as breast cancer (see Chapter 9).

- After menopause, regular consumption of phytoestrogens can increase the level of estrogen-like substances in circulation but to a lesser degree than levels obtained with hormone replacement therapy.

- Estrogen-like soy isoflavones may not only reduce hot flashes but have been shown to protect arterial and bone health (see Chapters 6, 7 and 8).

- The lignans in flaxseed have an antiestrogenic action that may also be useful in the prevention of breast cancer.

PHYTOESTROGENS AND HOT FLASHES

In the aftermath of the Finnish team's observations of phytoestrogen consumption in Japanese women, several clinical research experts tested the effectiveness of soy in reducing hot flashes in menopausal women.

The first study was carried out at Australia's Brighton Medical Clinic. Sixty menopausal women who were experiencing at least 14 significant hot flashes per week were selected. For a three-month period they were asked to add to their daily diet 45 g (1/3 cup) of flour camouflaged in their food. Some were given soy flour, others wholewheat flour, but neither group was told which they had. By the end of the study period, those women who had been given soy flour noted a gradual reduction of 40% in their hot flashes.

Another study carried out at the Jerusalem University Hospital monitored 145 women suffering from hot flashes. Ninety-five women chosen at random from among the sample group were given a daily portion of 80 g of tofu, two glasses of soy beverage, 5 mL (1 tsp.)

of miso and 15 mL (1 tbs.) of once-ground flaxseed (the other source of phytoestrogens) for a 12-week period. The second group made no changes in its diet. At the end of the study, the women of the first group noted a more significant reduction of their hot flashes; some women experienced a remarkable effect after only a few days, while others experienced only mild reactions. After the study had ended, some of the members of this group experienced a recurrence of their hot flashes. The soy and flaxseed phytoestrogens had made a difference.

A three-month study of 104 women that was carried out in Bologna, Italy, also showed that adding 60 g of powdered soy protein to their diet could diminish hot flashes by 26% after three weeks and 45% by the end of the three-month study period.

The effect of phystoestrogens is now recognized.

After several attempts to control my own hot flashes (vitamin E supplements, looser clothing, a fan in my office, taking a hot bath in the morning rather than at night, etc.), I began to consume tofu every day. I noticed a distinct reduction, both in the intensity and frequency of hot flashes.

I now recommend to women who consult me for hot flashes to consume soy-rich foods every day. Many of them have noticed an improvement. Some have experienced an even stronger impact when they increased their soy intake.

FOODS THAT HELP; FOODS THAT DON'T
Some foods, such as alcoholic beverages, can actually stimulate hot flashes by increasing the quantity of estrogen in circulation. Other foods, like hot soup, rapidly increase body temperatures even though they have no direct effect on the estrogen cycle.

On the other hand, foods rich in boron, such as nuts, dried legumes and dried fruits as well as fruits and vegetables (see Table 9, page 54), indirectly help soothe hot flashes by stimulating estrogen circulation in the blood.

PATHWAYS TO A SOLUTION

1. Incorporate soy and flaxseed in your daily diet.

Ignore the prejudice of your friends and family when it comes to strange, new foods and make the two best sources of phytoestrogens — soy and flaxseed — a part of your daily food intake. You can take soy in beverage form; as tofu, tempeh, soy protein powder; as flour; as cooked or roasted soybeans; as miso (see Table 8, page 51); or in the form of prepared foods featuring tofu or other forms of soy (see Table 10, page 56). Flaxseed can be ground to a fine powder and sprinkled on your cereal, on yogurt or on Creamed Tofu with Fruit dessert (recipe page 47). It's well worth the small effort, and the side effects could hardly be better: lower blood levels of bad cholesterol (LDL), increased good cholesterol (HDL), increased bone density and prevention of breast cancer.

Include in your daily food intake:

- 15 mL (1 tbs.) of once-ground flaxseed
  and
- 100 g (approximately 3.5 oz.) of tofu and 45 mL (3 tbs.) of soy protein powder and 2 tbs. roasted soybeans or any other soy-based product that enables you to consume approximately 75 mg of soy isoflavones per day (see Table 11, page 59). Japanese women's diets can contain up to 200 mg daily.

Be patient; you'll need from three to six weeks before you feel a difference and begin to notice the beneficial effects. If results are faster, so much the better.

Remember that daily intake is essential to obtain the desired effect. Two servings of tofu per week are not enough.

My favourite breakfast is a dish of Creamed Tofu with Fruit. I am convinced that breakfast is one of the best times to eat soy, as it is the meal

least affected by a busy social or professional schedule. Lunch and dinner don't
always give us the same opportunity.

If creamed tofu is not to your taste, whip up a glass of Creamy Tofu
Milk (see recipe, page 48). Delicious!

You can also prepare a tasty tofu and peanut butter spread or simply
add soy protein (see recipes, also on page 48) to other foods. You can also:

- Use a soy beverage instead of milk on your cereals or in your soups.
  Several soy beverages are now fortified with calcium and vitamin D,
  which means you may replace milk without having to take calcium
  supplements.
- Use miso as a seasoning to replace salt in sauces and soups.
- Replace meat with grilled tempeh.
- Use the soy-based spreads found in your local health-food store or
  supermarket on a healthy wholewheat bread.
- Cook up Chinese-style soups with bouillon, finely chopped green
  onion and a handful of tofu cubes; flavour with garlic, grated fresh
  ginger and some lime juice.
- Mix equal quantities of silken tofu and fruit-flavoured yogurt and
  serve for dessert or as a snack with fresh fruit or a few toasted almonds.

See the bibliography for books offering more soy-based recipes, to help
you add variety to your menu. And relax: you can never really eat too
much of these foods.

Creamed Tofu with Fruit

In a food processor, liquefy one well-peeled orange, cut into
sections, and one sweet apple, quartered. Add 100 g (approx. 3 oz.)
of silken tofu, such as Mori-Nu or Kikkoman, 5 to 15 g (1 tsp. to
1 tbs.) once-ground flaxseeds, and 45 mL (3 tbs.) of freshly ground
oat flakes. Mix until a smooth, creamy consistency is obtained.
Yields one portion.

Creamed Avocado with Tofu
Mix 60 g of silken tofu with the flesh of half a ripe avocado, 15 mL
(1 tbs.) lemon juice, and finely minced chives. Yields one cup.

Creamy Tofu Milk
Combine equal quantities of fat-free or 1% milk and silken tofu in a
blender and blend until smooth. Pour this creamy milk over your
favourite breakfast cereal or over pieces of fresh fruit.

Peanut Butter and Tofu Spread
Mix equal quantities of tofu and natural peanut butter; season with a
few drops of maple syrup or honey. Spread on toast or use as a dip
with sliced fresh fruits. Keeps well in the refrigerator for approximately one week.

Soy Protein
Mix 30 to 60 mL (2 to 4 tbs.) of soy protein powder into a glass of
milk or a bowl of yogurt.

Fruity Tofu Beverage
In a blender, combine 200 mL (7 oz.) fresh or frozen unsweetened
strawberries or blueberries with 100 g (3 oz.) silken tofu, 15 to 30
mL (1 to 2 tbs.) honey and five ice cubes. Blend until smooth.
Serve cold. Yields 2 or 3 servings.

Exquisite Tofu Dip
In a food processor, combine a 12 oz. piece firm silken tofu, the
juice of one-half lemon, 20 mL (4 tsp.) Dijon mustard, 15 mL
(1 tbs.) red wine vinegar, 30 mL (2 tbs.) finely chopped fresh chives
and basil, salt and pepper to taste. Mix until smooth. You can serve
immediately with raw veggies, but it keeps well in the refrigerator
for approximately one week. Yields about 500 mL (2 cups).

▨ Vanilla-Tofu Sauce

In a food processor mix a 12-oz. piece of firm silken tofu, 15 mL
(1 tbs.) honey and 2 mL (1/2 tsp.) vanilla. Mix until smooth and
creamy. This sauce can be used instead of whipped or clotted cream
on fresh fruits, or as a cake frosting. You'll love the taste! Yields
about 500 mL (2 cups).

2. Cut back your alcohol consumption.

Don't blame your friends or the convivial atmosphere at the restaurant
if your body thermostat goes out of kilter at a meal where the wine is
flowing. Even a simple aperitif can touch off enough of a hot flash to
throw you off balance or make you feel ill at ease. Monitor your body's
reactions, and cut back your alcohol consumption.

3. Increase your intake of foods rich in boron.

Boron, like calcium, magnesium and iron, is a mineral. It belongs to the
family of nutrients whose functions are now recognized and considered
essential. Because its action resembles that of estrogen — though its
power is much more limited — boron can help keep hot flashes under
control. It also appears to inhibit daily calcium loss and may be a useful
ally in the fight against osteoporosis.

A daily intake of about 3 mg of boron seems to be sufficient for a positive impact on hot flashes and calcium retention (see Table 13, page 61).
As you can see, a menu rich in fruits and vegetables, and including moderate amounts of nuts and dried fruits, can provide the boron you need.

For a satisfactory dose of boron and isoflavones, try the Creamed Avocado with Tofu. It keeps well in the refrigerator and can be eaten as a dip
with vegetable sticks or as a purée with a main dish of poultry or seafood.

4. Consider vitamin E supplements.

I've received numerous accounts of the positive effect of vitamin E
supplements in reducing hot flashes. Despite the multitude of studies

on the role of vitamin E and its antioxidant activities at the cellular membrane level, none has explored its effect on hot flashes. However, several epidemiological studies have established a link between vitamin E supplements and a reduced risk of cardiovascular illness, a finding that may be of interest to women over 50. If you are already taking a supplement of 200 or 400 IU of vitamin E and you have not experienced any hot flashes, don't hesitate to keep it up, as this dose is unlikely to produce side effects. If you are taking doses of more than 400 IU, consult Chapter 10.

5. Should you be taking evening primrose oil?

Some women swear by evening primrose oil. The oil, which is extracted from the flower of the same name, contains a peculiar variety of fat, gamma-linolenic acid. This fat is a member of the omega-6 family of essential acids and performs several important functions in the human body. It is manufactured by the human organism itself from the fat we consume, but its production is hampered by unfavourable circumstances: too much saturated or hydrogenated fat, too much alcohol, a lack of vitamins and minerals, or aging. The process slows further as women grow older and occurs more rapidly than in men, irrespective of diet.

We now know that evening primrose oil, being rich in gamma-linolenic acid, promotes the production of prostoglandins, which play a positive role in female hormonal balance. Hence its use in soothing premenstrual discomfort.

Its action during menopause is less well understood. A study of hot flashes carried out in England several years ago revealed only one positive effect — on night sweats. Still, many women find that it helps them.

If you want to give it a try, take it with meals, not on an empty stomach. Begin with a small dose and increase gradually. Evening primrose oil can cause side effects such as nausea in some women.

> As you can see, phytoestrogens can lessen the impact of hot flashes.

TABLE 8
A thumbnail dictionary of soy

Product and description	Use
Frozen soy desserts: made with soy milk or soy-based yogurt **Note:** These products may contain large quantities of sugar.	Check label.
Miso: fermented soybean paste; rich in sodium (salt); 603 mg sodium/ 15 mL (1 tbs.)	Use miso as a salt or soy sauce substitute in cooking. Adds flavour to vegetables, grains, tofu, sauces and soups.
PVH sauce: sauce based on hydrolyzed vegetable protein (soy, corn, wheat), unfermented, with corn syrup, caramel and salt.	
Shoyu: ("soy sauce" in Japanese); soy mixture; may contain wheat protein unless marked otherwise.	
Soy beverage: liquid extracted from soaked, boiled, cooked, molded and pressed soybeans. Several varieties are now enriched with calcium and vitamin D (check label); 300 mg calcium/250 mL, 7.5 g protein/250 mL	Soy beverage is pasteurized and available in liquid form, fresh or UHT. Used like cow's milk, it is available in different flavours and in a light version. Also available in powder.
Soy cheese: made with soy beverage, tofu and soy proteins	Can be consumed as is or used in recipes.
Soy flour: roasted, finely ground soybeans	Soy flour may be used in small quantities in baked goods.

TABLE 8 cont'd
A thumbnail dictionary of soy

Product and description	Use
Soy granules: roasted soybeans ground into granules	Granules are used primarily by the food processing industry to add nutritive value to rice or other grains.
Soy lecithin: extracted from soy oil (1–3% lecithin)	Lecithin is used as a stabilizer, an antioxidant and as a crystallizer for commercial products and as an emulsifier for fat products. Lecithin is also available as a supplement.
Soy nuts: soaked soybeans that are then oil or air roasted. Texture similar to peanuts. 40 g protein/100 g	Whole or chopped soy nuts are sold salt-free or salted.
Soy protein concentrate: contains 65% of protein extracted from soybeans in flake form. Soy fibres are intact.	
Soy protein isolate: contains 90% of protein extracted from soybeans in flake form. SPI can be found in many protein supplements. 20 g protein/30 mL powder	SPI is used by the food processing industry to increase product shelf-life, improve food texture or as an emulsifier. It is also added to infant formula supplements and diet supplements.
Soy sauce: dark brown, salty liquid derived from the fermentation of soybeans. A sodium-rich	

TABLE 8 cont'd
A thumbnail dictionary of soy

Product and description	Use
condiment. 1,017 mL sodium/15 mL (1 tbs.). Contains no isoflavones.	
Tamari: (another type of "soy sauce" in Japanese); made primarily of soy; may contain hydrolyzed proteins.	
Tempeh: soy combined with a whole grain, usually rice or millet. Soybeans are soaked in water, then cooked. A fermenting agent is added and left to work. Fresh tempeh has a white crust similar to Brie or Camembert cheese. Tempeh is soft, with a mushroom-like flavour. 19 g protein/100 g	Tempeh must be cooked before eating. Tasty as a main dish or snack if marinated for 20 minutes Add to spaghetti sauces, chili or soups. Steamed and grated, it can be mixed with mayonnaise in sandwiches.
Teriyaki: soy sauce flavoured with sugar, vinegar and spices.	
Tofu: soy liquid heated, curdled using a coagulant, then pressed into blocks. Tofu is white with a porous texture that allows it to absorb the flavours of sauces or other foods with which it is combined. 8 g protein/100 g ordinary soft tofu; 16 g protein/100 g ordinary firm tofu; 7 g protein/100 g silken tofu **Note:** light or low-fat tofu contains fewer isoflavones than other firm or extra-firm tofus.	Ready to eat, tofu needs no cooking. Ordinary tofu (soft or firm): sliced or cubed, in stews; used chopped to replace ground meat. Silken tofu (soft or firm), also called Japanese tofu, is ideal for dips, soups or fruit creams.

TABLE 9
Boron content of selected foods

Food	Portion		Boron (mg)
FRUITS AND VEGETABLES			
Avocado	1/2	1/2	2.1
Prunes	50 g	4 tbs.	0.9
Peach, dried	40 g	4 tbs.	0.8
Prune juice	125 mL	1/2 cup	0.8
Raisins	15 g	2 tbs.	0.7
Peach	1		0.6
Apricots, dried	3		0.5
Red grapes	90 g	1 cup	0.5
Pear	1		0.5
Plums	2		0.5
Dates	4		0.4
Orange	1		0.3
Apple	1		0.3
Celery	60 g	1/2 cup	0.3
Figs, dried	2		0.3
Kiwi fruit	1		0.3
Apple juice	125 mL	1/2 cup	0.3
Carrot	1		0.2
Broccoli	50 g	1/4 cup	0.2
Potato	1 small		0.1
SOURCES OF PROTEIN			
Red kidney beans, cooked	180 g	1 cup	2.6
Borlotto beans	180 g	1 cup	2.3
Lentils, cooked	180 g	1 cup	1.5
Chick peas, cooked	180 g	1 cup	1.2
Hazelnuts	20 g	2 tbs.	0.9
Almonds	20 g	2 tbs.	0.6
Peanut butter	15 mL	1 tbs.	0.4
Brazil nuts	5 medium		0.3

TABLE 9 cont'd
Boron content of selected foods

Food	Portion		Boron (mg)
	SOURCES OF PROTEIN CONT'D		
Walnuts	20 g	2 tbs.	0.2
	OTHER		
Red wine	100 mL	3 oz.	0.9
White wine	100 mL	3 oz.	0.3

TABLE 10
Soy-based foods, prepared dishes

Food	Soy product
AVAILABLE IN SPECIALTY STORES	
Tofu Caesar sandwich	Tofu
Tofu spaghetti sauce	Tofu
Tamari-mustard or tamari-peanut salad dressing	Soybeans
Salad dressing (5 flavours)	Tofu and miso
Mayonnaise	Silken tofu or soy beverage
Soy flakes	Soybeans
Dehydrated noodle soup (several varieties available)	Soybeans, miso
Vegetable soup	Miso
Scrambled tofu (imitation scrambled eggs)	Tofu
Instant soup mix	Soybean vegetable protein
Tofu burger	Tofu
Soy beverage (chocolate or vanilla)	Soy milk
Energy bar (wide variety on sale)	Soy protein isolate
Tofu cheeses	Tofu
Seasoning for poultry, eggs, pasta (dehydrated, in packet)	Tofu
Smoked, herbed tofu	Tofu
Tofu noodles	Tofu
Vegetarian paté	Tofu or soybeans
Grated Parmesan tofu	Tofu
Soy yogurt	Soybeans
Lasagna (soy noodles)	Tofu
Meatball stew, shepherd's pie	Soy protein
Tofu fricassee	Tofu

TABLE 10 cont'd
Soy-based foods, prepared dishes

Food	Soy product
SOY BEVERAGES	
Algae paté	Soy beverage
Leek paté	Organic soy beverage
Vegetable paté	Organic soy beverage
Leek quiche	Organic soy beverage, tofu
Millet pie	Soy beverage, tofu
Seitan pie	Soy beverage
"Meat" pie	Soy beverage, tofu
Vegetable rolls	Soy beverage
Vegetarian paté	Organic soy beverage, tofu
Galantine	Tofu
Firm or silken tofu	
Tempeh	
Ginger paté	Organic soy beverage, tofu
3-pepper paté	Organic soy beverage, tofu
Dijonnaise sauce	Organic soy protein
Terrine	Tofu
Vegetable dip	Organic soy beverage
Dressing for cabbage salad	Organic soy beverage
Cookies	Organic soy beverage
Yule log	Organic soy beverage
Maple cream-puffs	Organic soy beverage
Poppy-seed cake	Organic soy beverage
Soy cake	Organic soy beverage
Sweet cakes (several kinds)	Organic soy beverage
Maple, chocolate or coffee mousse	Organic soy beverage
Lemon, pumpkin pies	Organic soy beverage
Tapioca pudding	Organic soy beverage
Raisin brioche	Soy beverage
Wheat croissant	Soy beverage

TABLE 10 cont'd

Soy-based foods, prepared dishes

Food	Soy product
SOY BEVERAGES CONT'D	
Almond bread	Soy beverage
Carob bread	Soy beverage
AVAILABLE IN SUPERMARKETS	
Terrine	Organic tofu
Millet pie	Tofu
Tofu spread	Tofu
Soy beverages	
Natural or herbed tofu	Tofu
Meatless meatloaf	Soy protein products
Luncheon sausages	Soy protein isolate
Hot dogs	Soy protein isolate
"Garden style" cutlets	Soy protein isolate
Deli slices	Soy protein isolate
Veggie burger	Soy protein products
Chili sausages	Soy protein isolate

TABLE 11

Isoflavone* content of selected soy products**

Food	Portion	Isoflavones (mg)
Soy flour, full fat	50 g (1/2 cup)	84
Soy flour, fat removed	50 g (1/2 cup)	64
Tempeh, cooked	100 g (3.5 oz.)	50
Soybeans, cooked	50 g (1/2 cup)	49
Soybeans, roasted	30 g (4 tbs.)	35
Soybean chips	60 g (1 bag)	32
Tofu, silken type, firm	100 g (3.5 oz.)	27–29
Tempeh burger	100 g (3.5 oz.)	26
Tofu yogurt	175 g (3/4 cup)	26
Soy milk	250 mL (1 cup)	26
Regular tofu	100 g (3.5 oz.)	21
Soybean flakes, full fat	15 g	19
Soybean flakes, fat removed	15 g	18
Soy protein isolate	15 mL (1 tbs.)	11
Miso	5 mL (1 tsp.)	5
Soy sauce or tamari	5 mL (1 tsp.)	0
Soy oil	5 mL (1 tsp.)	0

* These values represent amounts of the most commonly measured types of isoflavones, genestein and daidzein.

** Isoflavone content of soy products can vary depending on the variety of soy, the crop year, the location, the process and the brand. This chart provides figures obtained from the latest series of analysis compiled by USDA–Iowa State University Database 1999.

TABLE 12

Three menus containing more than
75 mg of isoflavones* per day

Meal	1	2	3
Breakfast	Fruit juice	Fresh fruit	**Tofu-fruit drink**
	Creamed Tofu	Whole grain cereal	Wholewheat
	with Fruit**	**Creamy Tofu Milk****	bread
Lunch	Shredded chicken	Baked trout	Lentil soup
	Fresh vegetables	Cabbage with lemon	Raw vegetables
	Homemade dressing	Brown rice with	**Tofu Dip****
	Wholewheat bread	chives	Cheese cubes
	Fresh fruit	1/4 cantaloupe	with pita
			Applesauce
Snack	Milk and **soy protein**	**Roasted soybeans**	Yogurt and
			soy protein
Dinner	Wholewheat pasta	Health salad	Stir-fried shrimp
	Primavera sauce	(chick peas, feta,	with seasonal
	Spinach salad	tomato, green pepper,	vegetables
	Yogurt	romaine lettuce,	Brown rice with
	Fruit and **roasted**	salad dressing)	parsley
	soybeans	Fruits	Endive salad
		Vanilla–Tofu	Figs, clementines
		Sauce**	

* Foods shown in boldface type contain high doses of isoflavones.
** See pages 47–49 for recipes.

TABLE 13

A menu containing approx. 3 mg of boron*

Meal	Food	Quantity of boron
Breakfast	**Prune juice** 125 mL (1/2 cup)	0.8 mg
	1 slice toast with 15 mL (1 tbs.)	0.4 mg
	peanut butter	
	Milk and cereal	—
	Coffee	—
Snack	**Kiwi fruit** and 20 g (2 tbs.) **almonds**	0.9 mg
Lunch	Vegetable juice	—
	Chicken salad (chicken, young	0.25 mg
	lettuce, **celery**, **carrot**, with homemade	
	salad dressing)	
	Plain yogurt and **4 dates**	0.4 mg
Snack	**Apple**	0.32 mg
Dinner	Grilled salmon	—
	Cooked broccoli 80 g (1/2 cup)	0.23 mg
	Wholewheat bread	—
	Small green salad	—
	Fresh fruit	—
Snack	1 glass of milk	—
		Total: 3.3 mg

* Boldface type indicates foods rich in boron.

V

Bloating

Did you ever have the sudden sensation, an hour or two after a meal, that you've swallowed a beach ball? Even if the symptoms end a couple of hours later, or the next day, you've still got that uncomfortable feeling — or worse, considering the extra centimetres that have just appeared around your waist. It can happen any time, menopause specialists tell us; bloating is one of the most frequently reported discomforts women face.

The scientific literature is relatively silent on the subject. After all, this is hardly a condition that is likely to shorten your life. But at our nutrition clinic, we take a different approach. For us, it's a serious matter. Your diet may be the cause — and may contain the solution.

Some women become bloated when bowel movements become irregular. In fact, women are more prone to constipation than men, even more so with age. At menopause, the problem can become even more troublesome. Women need to fight more actively against what we call the lazy bowel syndrome.

Other women eat too much sugar without even noticing it, a cookie here and a chocolate there. . . . Regular intake of food with a high sugar content naturally causes a certain degree of intestinal fermentation that can result in bloating. Nothing to worry about, but it can be downright unpleasant.

Still others wolf down their daily sandwich or plate of pasta at lunch only to see their waistline expand an hour later.

Then there are the women who increase their milk intake in an effort to boost calcium and protect their bones against osteoporosis, but unknowingly develop a lactose intolerance. When this happens, bloating is accompanied by stomach cramps and diarrhea. As soon as lactose is eliminated from the diet, everything returns to normal.

Finally, bloating in some women may be related to an inflammatory disease of the digestive tract. This kind of problem is serious, and far less frequent than the preceding cases. It calls for a full-scale medical examination.

PATHWAYS TO A SOLUTION
Switching to elastic waistbands in your skirts and slacks can bring short-term relief, but only reviewing and improving your eating habits will really help you in the long run.

1. Solve your constipation problems.
Irregular bowel movements can do more than just cause bloating; they can negatively affect the liver function and the function of the digestive tract as a whole. You must not allow this kind of situation to develop.

As a first step, take a close look at your morning habits. Drink a glass of water when you get up, and eat at least a small amount of fibre-rich food soon afterwards; for example, fresh fruit, bran cereal, a bowl of yogurt or Creamed Tofu with Fruit (see recipe, page 47). Take a short break after this first meal. Nothing aggravates constipation more than leaving in a rush for a busy morning.

As a second step, evaluate your usual dietary fibre consumption (see Table 14, page 67), and if necessary, gradually increase your daily intake until you've reached 30 g per day. Take it easy; abrupt changes may only worsen the problem. At the same time, increase your water consumption to about two litres (eight glasses) a day to prevent dehydration. If, after a few weeks, your body cannot cope with the extra raw fruits, vegetables and fibre-rich cereal products, try a psyllium-based medication available without a prescription (such as Metamucil or Prodiem). It may help.

As a third step, increase your physical activity. Walking, dancing or any other kind of exercise stimulates the bowel and improves the intestinal function. Look for reasons to do things on foot: climb the subway stairs, park your car far from your destination and walk, adopt a dog, join a walking club, ride a bicycle, or pull on those new in-line skates. Make physical activity an integral part of your new health routine.

2. Watch your sugar consumption.

Sugar in any form is a fermentation agent. To check whether this kind of fermentation coincides with your bloating, write down the foods you eat for several days, underlining those that contain sugar in appreciable amounts: cookies, jams and jellies, honey, maple syrup, cream-rich desserts, pies, cakes, soft drinks, raisins, dates, chewing gum, chocolates or mints. If you eat any of these foods on any given day, eliminate them completely from your diet for several days and note the difference. Replace jams with applesauce or a sliced banana, sugary desserts with fresh fruit or fruit salad, dried fruits with almonds or pistachios. The aim is not to lose weight, but simply to cut down on bloating by reducing your intake of sweets.

3. Cut back on your bread or pasta consumption at lunchtime.

In my experience, many women complain of serious bloating despite eating a balanced diet. The following example seems typical.

Francine, age 48, has just begun her menopause. She consulted me after putting on 4.5 kg (10 lb.) in six months; now, daily bloating has created an unbearable situation. Her diet is next to perfect: three meals a day with a judicious choice of foods and a limited amount of calories. Her daily exercise was quite sufficient. After close evaluation of her menu, I suggested ways of reducing the intake of carbohydrate at noon, replacing her midday sandwich with a good source of proteins and a few raw or cooked vegetables. Result: the bloating disappeared rapidly and Francine lost 3.4 kg (7 lb.) in four months thanks to a handful of other minor changes in diet.

To avoid bread or pasta at midday, choose instead:

- a chicken breast accompanied by a fresh green salad and dressing;
- tuna or shrimp salad with a few slices of avocado;
- a bean-based soup, raw vegetables and cottage or ricotta cheese;
- a bean or lentil salad, fresh vegetables and yogurt;
- broiled meat, poultry or fish with plenty of steamed vegetables.

Not long after you adopt a menu like this, see how you feel. If you're feeling better and your tummy has kept within its normal dimensions, try adding bread or pasta to your menu. Chances are you'll nail the true culprit.

4. Eliminate or diminish your lactose consumption.

Lactose is a sugar that occurs naturally in fresh dairy products such as milk, yogurt, cottage cheese and ice cream (see Table 15, page 68). It can be digested thanks to an enzyme called lactase that is normally produced in the intestine. If this enzyme is deficient, you may experience cramps, bloating or diarrhea after eating milk products. If the

diarrhea becomes chronic, absorption of certain key nutrients is significantly reduced.

If you are experiencing this kind of problem, eliminate from your
diet all sources of lactose for at least two weeks, and note any changes
that occur. After two weeks, drink a large glass of milk and observe how
your body reacts. If the symptoms reappear immediately, change your
diet routine to include the smallest possible quantity of lactose. You
may, however, use milks whose lactose has been predigested (products
such as Lactaid and Lacteeze), or take Lactaid or Lactrase tablets before
eating a lactose-rich dairy product. If these steps only partially solve
the problem, avoid foods that contain lactose altogether. You should,
however, look for other sources of calcium and include a vitamin D
supplement to protect your bones.

5. If these measures do not produce results, consult your physician for a more extensive examination.

Several illnesses of the digestive tract present similar symptoms: extreme
fatigue, low iron in the blood, acute diarrhea or constipation and, of
course, bloating. These symptoms may be the sign of inflammatory
diseases of the bowel, of an irritable colon, of diverticulitis or celiac disease. All can be identified and diagnosed with specialized tests. These
are serious conditions with specific dietary requirements, so if you
experience any of the symptoms described above, I advise you to first
consult your physician and then see a dietitian to modify your food
intake accordingly.

> You can quickly solve your bloating problems by paying closer
> attention to your fibre, sugar, carbohydrate or lactose intake.
> Don't delay one day longer.

TABLE 14
Food fibre sources

Food	Portion		Fibre (g)
FRUITS AND VEGETABLES			
Avocado	1/2	1/2	9
Raspberry	120 g	1 cup	8
Mango	170 g	1 cup	6
Pear	1	1	5
Potato with peel, baked	1	1	5
Blueberries or strawberries	150 g	1 cup	4
Corn or green peas, cooked	80 g	1/2 cup	4
Kiwi fruit, apple, orange	1	1	3
Fresh apricots	3	3	2
Banana, fresh fig	1	1	2
Carrot	1	1	2
CEREAL PRODUCTS			
Bran cereal with psyllium	20 g	1/4 cup	8
Pot barley, cooked	100 g	1 cup	5
Wheat bran cereal	20 g	1/4 cup	5
Wheat bran	15 g	1/4 cup	4
Brown rice, cooked	190 g	1 cup	3
Wheat germ	30 g	1/4 cup	3
Wholewheat pasta	140 g	1 cup	2
Wholewheat bread	1 slice	1 slice	1
PROTEIN SOURCES			
Lima beans, cooked	180 g	1 cup	16
Red kidney beans, cooked	180 g	1 cup	15
Black beans, cooked	180 g	1 cup	15
Lentils, chick peas, cooked	180 g	1 cup	10
Almonds	30 g	2 tbs.	3
Peanut butter	30 mL	2 tbs.	2
Regular tofu, firm	125 g	4 oz.	2

TABLE 15

Lactose* content of several foods

Food	Portion	Lactose (g)
MILK AND MILK DERIVATIVES		
Whole milk	250 mL (1 cup)	11
Lactose-free milk (Lactaid or Lacteeze)	250 mL (1 cup)	0.05 or less
Yogurt	125 g (1/2 cup)	2.5
CHEESE		
Hard cheese	30 g (1 oz.)	0.4–0.7
Fresh cheese (cottage, ricotta)	120 g (1/2 cup)	4
Lactose-free cheese	30 g (1 oz.)	less than 0.01%
MILK-BASED DESSERTS		
Ice cream or ice milk	125 mL (1/2 cup)	5

* Several medications also contain small amounts of lactose. If contents are not shown on label, ask your pharmacist.

VI

Protecting
Your Arteries

*F*or years, heart disease was considered a man's illness. But women are not immune. It affects both sexes but the symptoms appear in women about 10 years later. In fact, heart disease is our leading cause of death. However, even though it's true that heart disease kills more women than breast cancer does, we cannot say the same thing about menopausal women. The death rate for women between 50 and 60 is three times higher from cancer than from cardiovascular disease; the incidence of death from cardiovascular disease begins to rise only after age 70 (see Table 16, page 81).

Still, the risk of heart failure is two to three times greater after menopause than before. Better face facts: an ounce of prevention is worth a pound of cure.

Now, the good news: between 1979 and 1995, the death rate from heart disease among Canadian women dropped by 36%.

A WOMAN'S HEART IS DIFFERENT

Until menopause, a woman seems to be protected against heart disease. She has less "bad" cholesterol (LDL) and much more "good" cholesterol (HDL) in her blood than a man of the same age. In other words, she benefits more from the HDL, which clears the excess cholesterol accumulated in the arteries and carries it to the liver where it can be excreted in the bile.

With the onset of menopause, a woman experiences cholesterol problems for the first time. From pre- to post-menopause, total cholesterol increases by an average of 1.1 micromol (mmol) (20%) over an eight-year period. For example, a 45-year-old woman with a total cholesterol of 5.1 mmol could well register 6.2 mmol at age 53.

During the same period, triglycerides (another kind of fat circulating in the blood) increase and blood pressure rises. The protection women enjoyed during their years of menstruation disappears.

Despite the changes associated with menopause, women's hearts continue to share common traits with men's. In both sexes, the risk of heart attack or stroke increases with smoking, high blood pressure, high blood cholesterol, a sedentary lifestyle and excess weight.

But other risk factors are different. Unlike men, women's fasting insulin levels increase with age, making them more susceptible to diabetes. Worse, the risk of cardiovascular complications is twice as great among women suffering from diabetes as compared with men. A woman whose good cholesterol (HDL) level is lower than average, or whose triglyceride level is higher than average, is also more vulnerable than a man with comparable levels.

Symptoms are different too. A woman may occasionally experience shortness of breath, nausea and the occasional pain in the arms, chest or jaw before she has a heart attack. In men, intense chest pain accompanies the heart attack.

A QUESTION OF HORMONES?

In the late 1950s a number of research teams, noting that women, prior to menopause, were protected from cardiovascular disease, set out to verify the protective effect of estrogen on the heart and arteries. Convinced that estrogen could be *the* solution to cardiac problems, some researchers gave men high doses of the female hormone but obtained unsatisfactory results. On the other hand, some studies have shown that taking estrogen after menopause could improve cholesterol levels and blood vessel elasticity without necessarily eliminating other risk factors such as high blood pressure and triglyceride levels. Furthermore, when progesterone was added, the protective effect was decreased and varied according to the type of progesterone used.

Before we conclude that hormones are *the* answer, we might well ask ourselves why the heart disease frequency in women does not rise until 20 years after the estrogen in the body declines. How can we also explain why plump women, who produce more estrogen in their fat tissue, are more at risk of heart disease than slender women?

Most of these questions, and others, still remain unanswered, and until very recently, no study had adequately assessed the impact of hormone replacement therapy on cardiac mortality, the crucial issue.

However, the Heart and Estrogen/Progestin Replacement Study (HERS), a clinical trial involving 2,763 women with established coronary disease (a past infarctus, bypass surgery or angioplasty), showed that hormone replacement therapy did not reduce the overall risk of death from cardiovascular disease. The investigators from some 20 university research centres in the United States concluded that treatment with hormones (estrogen and progesterone) can improve cholesterol levels but does not reduce the overall rate of cardiac events among postmenopausal women with established coronary disease. The authors added that based on their findings, they did not recommend prescribing hormones to prevent heart disease among women at risk. Published in the *American Medical Association Journal* in August 1998, the study clearly shows that the hormone-heart hypothesis is not yet conclusive.

More definitive answers about the real cardiovascular benefits of hormonal treatment for women in good health will become available in

2005 when the Women's Health Initiative Randomized Trial, a study coordinated by the National Institutes of Health in Washington, reaches its conclusion.

A QUESTION OF DIET AND LIFESTYLE?

According to Dr. Elizabeth Barrett-Connor, who coordinated the PEPI trial, another major research project on women at menopause, the actual difference in the incidence of heart disease between women in Japan and women in the United States is greater than between women who take hormones and those who do not. In other words, lifestyle may have a greater impact than hormones do. That is why Dr. Barrett-Connor points to the significant role played by nutrition, smoking and physical activity.

Though numerous studies have examined the effect of nutrition on cardiovascular health in men, few have focused on women. One of the most fascinating trials was conducted in Scandinavia over a 12-year period with 1,400 women between the ages of 40 and 64. The authors, who believed they had found a connection between the incidence of heart attack and obesity or the intake of fat, discovered instead that there was a link with a low food and calorie intake. They concluded that the cardiovascular problems in this population might be attributed to a lack of protective nutrients.

The Nurses' Health Study, a survey conducted since 1980 on 80,000 American nurses, also outlines the role of diet in heart disease. During the first 14 years of the study, researchers from the Harvard School of Public Health observed 939 incidents of cardiovascular illness (non-fatal myocardial infarction or death by coronary disease), but failed to establish any correlation with total fat consumption. They noted instead that the risk of cardiac disease rose by 21% with each addition of 2.3 g of hydrogenated fat (trans fatty acid) in the participants' diet.

Another team of investigators reexamined the diet in The Nurses' Health Study and observed that frequent nut consumption (approximately 5 oz. per week) was associated with a lower risk of heart disease;

they also looked at fatal versus non-fatal coronary disease and saw that a higher intake of alpha-linolenic acid (the kind of fat found in fish, flaxseeds, walnuts and canola oil) seemed protective against fatal infarctus.

ARE YOU VULNERABLE?

You won't be awakened at night by a gradual clogging of your arteries, or by excess blood cholesterol. But by the time pains in your chest or your left arm begin to worry you, it may be too late. Don't wait until that happens to find out if you are at risk.

Your family history is the first factor to consider. If a parent, grandparent, uncle or aunt has suffered a cardiovascular illness or had a major operation before age 60, you are more vulnerable.

Your lifestyle is also a factor.

If you smoke 35 cigarettes a day, you run a seven to 10 times greater risk than if you are a non-smoker. Smoking nullifies the protection provided by estrogen, lowers the good cholesterol (HDL) and increases the platelets responsible for blood coagulation. Two-thirds of early heart attacks suffered by women under 50 occur in smokers.

The less regular physical activity you engage in, the greater the risk. If you easily succumb to fried foods, if you can't resist crackers, cookies and potato chips, if you consume plenty of meat and cheese, if you must have butter or margarine on your bread, your intake of saturated and hydrogenated fats increases your risk.

Excess weight can be harmful. If your waistline is greater than 85 cm (33 in.), excess weight under your belt increases triglycerides and bad cholesterol and lowers good cholesterol.

If you suffer from **diabetes** or **high blood pressure**, your risk is greater. But don't be discouraged. By improving your lifestyle, you can lessen the effects of your condition.

However, if you suffer from low blood sugar or hypoglycemia, watch what you eat — but don't lose any sleep. Your arteries may not be affected.

Tests to complete your assessment

A **lipid profile** can give you more information. Even if your family history is a cause for concern, you may have a clean bill of health. Get a referral for a full battery of tests to find out the levels of *total* cholesterol, *HDL* (good cholesterol), *LDL* (bad cholesterol) and triglycerides; these blood tests will give you a complete lipid profile. When you get the results, don't worry too much about your total cholesterol level, which reveals only a partial picture; calculate your risk factor (as indicated below) to get the overall picture.

> To determine your cardiovascular risk factor, simply divide your total cholesterol by your HDL. For example: if your total cholesterol is 7.3 mmol and your HDL is 1.5 mmol, divide 7.3 by 1.5. Your risk factor is 4.8.
>
> If your risk factor is 4.5 or less, rest easy. But if your risk factor is 4.6 or greater, you should try to make changes in your lifestyle, as suggested in Pathways to a Solution (see page 75).

A **homocysteine level test** may help complete the information. If your risk factor is under 4.5, but you are still concerned about your family history and lifestyle, ask for a blood *homocysteine* level test. A high homocysteine level may reveal clogged arteries even if your cholesterol level is normal. If the analysis shows a normal homocysteine level — about 10 mmol/L — there is no cause for concern; your cardiovascular risk factors are low. If your homocysteine level exceeds 14 mmol/L, your risk of heart failure is three times higher.

> *Homocysteine* is an amino acid that helps produce certain proteins in the body. It is always present in the blood, but becomes fully active only when it receives sufficient amounts of three B vitamins: folic acid, pyridoxine (B6) and B12. When a diet is deficient in these vitamins, homocysteine accumulates in the blood, contributes to the thickening of the artery walls, and

heightens the risk of clot formation by increasing the adhesiveness of blood plaque. Greater intake of folic acid (see Table 17, page 82) through food and supplements can lower homocysteine levels.

A **fasting insulin measurement** is another test that helps predict future problems. If you have excess fat around your waist, a fasting insulin level analysis will make it possible to predict a few years in advance whether you are heading toward diabetes. When the fasting insulin level increases, insulin becomes less and less efficient, and must be produced in increasing quantities to perform the same tasks; this is known as insulin resistance. Things go from bad to worse: increased insulin or insulin resistance lowers sugar tolerance; diminished sugar tolerance leads to type II diabetes. This common post-menopausal condition multiplies five- or six-fold the risk of cardiovascular disease.

If your fasting insulin level is high, you can change your lifestyle to delay the onset of these problems.

Note: Not all laboratories carry out homocysteine or fasting insulin level tests, but they are becoming more and more available.

PATHWAYS TO A SOLUTION

If several risk factors are present, move quickly to take the steps listed below: they can increase your good cholesterol (HDL), and lower your bad cholesterol (LDL), blood pressure and fasting insulin levels. A 0.25-mmol increase in HDL can reduce the risk by 50%. You may even lose a few pounds and hardly notice it, and your cardiovascular health will gradually improve.

If you have no risk factors, but want to prevent cardiac problems and ensure overall health, take appropriate steps to cultivate healthy arteries over the long term.

1. Focus on the quality of the fats.

Studies conducted over recent years have established clearly that there are good fats and bad fats; good fats protect the health of the arteries, reduce bad cholesterol and may even reduce the likelihood of fatal coronary events; bad fats have the opposite effect. To minimize the risks of having a coronary illness, focus more than ever on the good fats.

Foods rich in *monounsaturated* fats belong to this group. They protect good cholesterol, reduce bad cholesterol, and even help control diabetes. They are mainly found in extra-virgin olive oil, canola oil, hazelnut oil, avocados, olives, almonds and pistachios.

Foods rich in *omega-3* fats also have a marvellous effect on cardiovascular health; their action on blood platelets is similar to that of aspirin, and limits the possibility of blood clots. Better still, they lower triglyceride levels, can diminish arrhythmia in some cardiac patients, and even reduce the risk of fatal coronary events. Among the foods rich in omega-3 fats are all fish, especially fat fish like salmon, mackerel and sardines. Flaxseed, walnuts, soy and canola contain substantial quantities. Dark green, leafy vegetables like spinach, Swiss chard, dandelion leaves, collards and kale have small amounts.

French researchers in Lyon, under the direction of Michel de Lorgeril, have provided the most striking demonstration yet of the benefits of good fats. These doctors monitored 605 cardiac patients who had suffered a heart attack. For more than 46 months, they reduced the meat intake of half of the patients and put special emphasis on foods rich in omega-3 fats and on fruits and vegetables, without setting strict limits to the quantities to be consumed. With this diet, known as the Mediterranean diet, the researchers managed to reduce the mortality rate and number of second heart attacks by 70% compared with the control group, an achievement that surpasses all other interventions involving lipid-lowering medication.

Foods rich in *bad* fats, beginning with the *saturated* fats found in meat, eggs, cream and cheese, increase the bad cholesterol (LDL). Without avoiding them completely, you can easily reduce your intake by rationing your portions of meat, forgetting to butter your bread, sampling fine cheese less frequently and reserving cream for very special occasions.

Foods rich in *hydrogenated* fats increase cardiovascular risk even more dramatically. Such fats turn up just about everywhere: in many baked foods, fast foods, potato chips, crackers, cookies, most margarine and other processed foods. Read the label closely, and avoid foods that include hydrogenated fats or shortening on the list of ingredients.

2. Don't let all fats frighten you.

The Mediterranean diet, which is rich in good fats, looks like a much more promising way to promote cardiovascular health than declaring an all-out war on all fats, as Americans have been doing for the last several years. The war on fat may even be producing the opposite effect. A recent study that compared the effects of two diets on cardiovascular risk factors in menopausal women was an eye-opener for many. The first diet contained less fat and more starchy food, while the second had a higher content of good fats and a lighter content of starches. The researchers were astonished to note that the first diet contributed to higher triglyceride and fasting insulin levels in addition to a reduction of good cholesterol (HDL), but the second diet did not increase these risk factors.

Instead of avoiding all fats, eat *good* fats in moderation. Instead of using salad dressings that have no oil or are low in calories, make your own with extra-virgin olive oil or canola oil; eat fatty fish like trout, salmon or sardines regularly; for snacks, reach for walnuts or almonds instead of crackers or cookies full of hydrogenated fats. The right foods can protect your arteries.

3. Increase your soy consumption.

In the summer of 1995, the results of 29 studies that used soy to lower cholesterol surprised many *New England Journal of Medicine* readers. People who made soy a part of their daily diet saw their bad cholesterol decrease by 13%, their triglycerides decline by 10.5% and their good cholesterol rise by 2.4% even though, in the majority of cases, the same people had consumed as much fat, saturated fat, cholesterol and calories as those who had not taken soy. People with high levels of cholesterol (8.6 mmol) achieved reductions of nearly 20% by eating two to three servings of soy-rich food every day. Of course, the soy was rich in isoflavones, the phytoestrogen described in Chapter 4 and listed in Table 11, page 59.

At the Baker Medical Research Institute in Melbourne, Australia, researchers set out to assess the effect of soy isoflavones not only on cholesterol, but also on the arterial health of some 20 women. They reported that taking 80 mg of isoflavones from soy per day for five to six weeks improved arterial wall elasticity, although this elasticity normally declines with age. The authors even likened this improvement to the results obtained with hormone replacement therapy.

To get the full benefit of soy, make it part of your daily diet in the form of tofu (see recipe ideas on pages 47–49), soy beverage or soy protein isolate. A daily intake of 75 to 100 mg of isoflavones can do wonders for your arteries (see Table 12, page 60).

4. Increase your consumption of soluble fibres.
Unlike *insoluble* fibres found in wheat bran, which increase fecal volume and prevent constipation, *soluble* fibres (found in legumes, oat bran, psyllium, pot barley, rice or corn bran, apples and other fruits and vegetables) promote the excretion of cholesterol in the bile and intestines. A few meals a week with lentils or chick peas, a bowl of psyllium-enriched cereal several times a week, an apple at snack time, and a salad at noon are changes you can easily make to help lower your cholesterol level.

Furthermore, a diet abundant in fruits and vegetables — up to seven or eight portions a day — substantially increases your intake of antioxidants, your reserves of vitamin C, carotenoids, potassium and magnesium, and helps to lower blood pressure, another significant risk factor.

5. Take the appropriate supplement, if necessary.
  • A supplement of vitamin B-complex
If your homocysteine level is too high, a vitamin B complex supplement taken every day should give you at least 400 µg of folic acid. The

additional dose of vitamin B can lower your homocysteine level and reduce this risk factor.

- A vitamin E supplement

Antioxidants like vitamin E can protect against the oxidation of bad cholesterol. A number of studies of various populations have associated high doses of vitamin E, taken as a supplement, with a significant reduction in the risk of cardiovascular disease and a slower progression of atherosclerosis. A supplement of 400 IU per day is an acceptable dose. Do not exceed this dose if you are already taking anticoagulants or if you suffer from high blood pressure or hyperthyroidism.

6. Don't cut out wine, but . . .

Wine lovers and people who enjoy life regard wine as an elixir. But caution is in order! Wine does not have a monopoly on nutritional assets. Of course, it contains polyphenols, which act as antioxidants and seem to increase good cholesterol.

But wine can be harmful to women suffering from hormone-dependent breast cancer. A study of menopausal women in the United States, Denmark and Portugal showed that moderate wine consumption raised blood estrogen levels.

Another study compared the effect of wine on menopausal women undergoing hormone replacement therapy with women who were not. Researchers at the Bringham and Women's Hospital in Boston observed that among a group of women who drank wine, blood estrogen levels were three times higher in women receiving hormone replacement therapy than in women who were not.

Despite all the claims and counter claims, a moderate intake for a woman should not exceed one glass of red or white wine a day.

7. Increase your physical activity.

Regular physical activity can increase good cholesterol (HDL), make insulin work more efficiently, lower the fibrinogen level (another risk factor) and slow blood coagulation! Who could ask for anything more?

To achieve these results, plan to do about 30 minutes of moderate exercise every day or almost every day. You don't have to become a jogging freak; just walk or go cycling, play golf, garden, or carry packages and take the stairs instead of the elevator. Make your muscles work regularly, and you will reap as many rewards as if you had stopped smoking.

> Protecting our arteries is a lifelong commitment. Adopt a daily program now. Chances are you'll live longer and feel better.

TABLE 16

Principal causes of death in women 50 and over

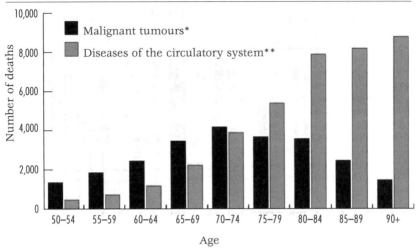

* Malignant tumours of the digestive system, the respiratory system, the breast, the cervix and the bladder.

** Principal diseases of the circulatory system are the following: myocardial infarctus (acute, old), angina, pericarditis, hypertensive diseases, cardiac insufficiency, cerebrovascular diseases and atherosclerosis.

Source: Statistics Canada, 1995

TABLE 17
Food sources of folic acid*

Food	Portion		Folic acid (µg)
FRUITS AND VEGETABLES			
Spinach, cooked	180 g	1 cup	277
Avocado	1	1	124
Asparagus, cooked	90 g	1/2 cup	88
Broccoli, cooked	160 g	1 cup	78
Romaine lettuce	60 g	1 cup	76
Orange juice	125 mL	1/2 cup	55
Green peas, cooked	80 g	1/2 cup	50
Brussels sprouts, cooked	80 g	1/2 cup	47
Orange	1	1	40
Kale, cooked	130 g	1 cup	30
Strawberries	150 g	1 cup	28
Grapefruit juice	125 mL	1/2 cup	26
Kiwi fruit	1	1	17
GRAIN PRODUCTS			
Soy flour	40 g	1/2 cup	147
Wheat germ	30 g	1/4 cup	80
Dark buckwheat flour	50 g	1/2 cup	63
Raisin Bran, Shreddies	50 g	1 cup	33
All Bran	20 g	1/4 cup	17
MEAT AND OTHER PROTEIN SOURCES			
Lentils, cooked	180 g	1 cup	378
Chick peas, cooked	180 g	1 cup	298
Calf liver, cooked	90 g	3 oz.	272
Black kidney beans, cooked	180 g	1 cup	256
Red kidney beans, cooked	180 g	1 cup	242
Beef liver, cooked	90 g	3 oz.	187
White kidney beans, cooked	180 g	1 cup	153
Soybeans, roasted	15 g	2 tbs.	44
Sunflower seeds	20 g	2 tbs.	38

TABLE 17 cont'd

Food sources of folic acid*

Food	Portion		Folic acid (µg)
MEAT AND OTHER PROTEIN SOURCES CONT'D			
Egg, cooked	1	1	23
Tofu, regular	125 g	1/2 cup	19
MILK PRODUCTS			
2% cottage cheese	225 g	1 cup	30
OTHER			
Torula yeast	8 g	1 tbs.	300

* Recommended nutritional intake: 185 µg/day, age 25–49
  (Canada 1990)   195 µg/day, age 50–74

VII

Preserving Your Bones

*D*on't take your bones for granted! They may seem solid enough to last a lifetime, but in fact bones are alive and vulnerable. Every day, through a process of breakdown and remodelling, our skeleton changes its composition. It reaches maximum strength when we are in our thirties, then begins to deteriorate during our forties. As a rule, we all lose bone tissue as we grow older, but the loss accelerates at menopause. If we let poor lifestyle habits harm our bones, remodelling lags behind, and bone loss becomes abnormally high. This condition is known as osteoporosis (see Chapter 8).

Before having a closer look at this disease that affects one woman in four, let's examine how bones function normally and go over the tools we can use to keep them strong for as long as possible.

BUILDING HEALTHY BONES

Many nutrients are vital to bone growth and maintenance. Calcium certainly plays a leading role, but other minerals and vitamins share the responsibility. Some of them work with calcium on bone growth; others promote bone density. Some factors, both nutritional and non-nutritional, help the body absorb bone-building materials; others help prevent losses.

Bone-building materials. Bone-building depends primarily on consumption of calcium-rich foods. The more dietary calcium we consumed during our growth period, the greater our bone density. Insufficient calcium intake during adolescence means thinner and more fragile bone tissue for life. In addition to calcium, substances such as zinc, manganese, copper and vitamins C and K also play an active role (see Tables 18 to 23, on pages 92 to 102).

Guardians of bone density. Maintaining good bone density is one of the best ways to prevent fractures. Women who regularly consume more vitamins C and K, zinc, magnesium and fibre have significantly higher vertebral bone density than those who neglect these nutrients. Women who eat plenty of fruits and vegetables not only obtain sufficient quantities of these vitamins and minerals; they also reduce the acidity of their bodies. This means they protect the mineral content of their bones.

Acidity, both in foods and in the body, is so poorly understood that it's worth a short paragraph. Many people mistakenly believe that eating acidic fruits like oranges, grapefruit and tomatoes releases acid into the body. In fact, quite the opposite occurs. When such fruits and vegetables are digested and absorbed, they reduce blood acidity and help protect bone calcium, according to several studies.

The allies of calcium absorption. The passage of calcium through the blood to the skeleton is neither simple nor straightforward. Many nutritional and non-nutritional factors are involved in the journey; some help and some hinder. Calcium's principal partners include vitamin D, estrogen, lactose, magnesium, fats and proteins (in sufficient quantities), and regular exercise. Among the main factors that impede calcium absorption are stress, disease, a sedentary lifestyle and certain medications (see Table 24, page 103). For optimal calcium absorption, you must not only ingest the right amount; you must also recruit as many allies as you can.

Additional losses. Your body does not retain all the calcium it has absorbed. Each day, it loses some calcium in the form of sweat, feces and urine. The urinary losses alone can amount to 100 to 250 mg of calcium a day. You can minimize these losses by paying attention to your salt and protein intake. See A Few Preventive Measures, pages 88 to 91.

OUR SKELETON'S DUAL ROLE

The first function of our skeleton is to support the body's muscles and soft tissue. The second is to act as a calcium storehouse whose primary responsibility is to meet the needs of the blood. What's at stake is bone solidity. When there is insufficient calcium in the blood, the bones supply the blood with calcium to allow the brain, lungs and muscles (including the heart muscle) to function. This rescue mission goes unnoticed until the day the calcium reserves in the bone drop to alarming levels.

Your blood calcium level can vary with diet. For example, when you eat too much protein and/or sugary food, you increase the acidity in your body. The excess acidity causes blood calcium to drop, and bone calcium must be used to restore the balance. If you seldom call on your calcium reserves, your skeleton will adapt, and won't be substantially weakened. But if you request calcium on a frequent basis, your bones will slowly but surely deteriorate.

THE STRENGTH OF OUR BONES

Skeletal strength depends on bone density, which in turn depends mainly on the calcium and vitamin D we've ingested during our growth period. The more calcium we have consumed while growing, the denser our bones will remain. In recent years, however, nutritional surveys have shown that few young women get a sufficient amount of calcium; as a result, many reach menopause with barely adequate bone density.

Total body weight also has an impact on skeletal strength; the more weight the skeleton must carry, the greater the bone density. This is why large-framed women have a greater bone mass and a lower fracture rate than slender women.

Bone strength also depends on the way we use our bones. A woman who uses her bones regularly will have stronger bones than her inactive counterpart. Your bones adapt to meet the demands you put on them. Just as you can strengthen your muscles, you can strengthen your bones. They grow stronger if they work to support the weight of your body every day or several times a week. If they are not used, they lose strength, due to lack of work!

I once had the good fortune to attend an osteoporosis workshop chaired by Dr. Robert Heaney. This international authority pointed out that *we have the bones we need*. It took me a few minutes to understand his remark, but I have not forgotten it. I learned that we have considerable control over the health of our bones and that using them regularly is a good way to strengthen them.

NORMAL BONE TISSUE LOSSES

Bone is living tissue in a perpetual state of remodelling. Until our mid-thirties, we accumulate more bone tissue in our skeleton than we lose. When we reach our forties, the depletion process outstrips remodelling. The bones undergo a slow, gradual loss resulting in a reduction of about 0.5 to 1% of the skeleton's mass per year. Losses increase:

- when your diet doesn't include enough calcium and other minerals and vitamins;
- when you aren't sufficiently physically active;
- when you smoke;
- when you are sick and/or bed-ridden;
- when you regularly take certain kinds of medication (Table 24, page 103).

A calcium level that falls below the World Health Organization (WHO) guidelines for a given age group signals an abnormal loss, which can lead to osteoporosis (see Chapter 8).

At menopause, another type of bone loss occurs. It is caused by a decline in estrogen. This kind of bone loss, which can amount to 3% of the skeletal mass per year for about five years, is not associated with nutrition or other lifestyle factors. It stabilizes with the end of the hormonal transition period.

A woman's bone density before menopause determines the impact of the loss caused by the hormonal change. A woman who has a good bone density at the onset of menopause may lose 15% of her bone mass and still have stronger bones at age 60 than a young woman who does not have good bone mass to begin with.

Even good nutrition cannot prevent losses due to menopause, but you can minimize the losses that come with lifestyle. The more good things you do for your bones and the younger you are when you do them, the more your skeleton will benefit. But it is never too late.

A FEW PREVENTIVE MEASURES

To prevent osteoporosis, look after your bones like the apple of your eye! No matter how old you are you can strengthen them. Some of the preventive measures listed below are quite similar to the suggestions for curing osteoporosis (see Chapter 8). To reach the recommended amounts of vitamins and minerals, try modifying your diet before turning to supplements; the situation is not as urgent as if you already had osteoporosis.

For women who have already consulted similar lists, this one may seem short; but it tells you all you need to know.

1. Increase your regular physical activity.

All studies point to one thing: physical activity is one of the key factors in maintaining a good bone structure. Nothing else is as beneficial.

Boston researchers studied some 40 women between ages 50 and 70.

Half followed an exercise program, attending twice-weekly classes of less than an hour; the other half remained sedentary. After a year, not only did the women who exercised have stronger bones, but they also had superior muscle mass. As one of the researchers remarked, the classic means for preventing osteoporosis (calcium, supplements and medication) improve bone quality, but only exercise can strengthen both the bones and the muscles.

Physical activity also has a beneficial effect on sleep habits. Some studies report that physically active people fall asleep on average in 15 minutes; sedentary people take 30 minutes and wake up less rested than active people. You can increase your physical activity even if exercise classes aren't your cup of tea. At every possible opportunity, use your legs and your muscles. Carry your packages instead of having them delivered; leave your car at home and use public transit; climb the stairs instead of taking the escalator or the elevator; plan your shopping so you'll have to walk for 10 to 15 minutes several times a week; ask a friend to join you on hikes in the city or the country; get involved in a sport you enjoy, even if you haven't done it for a few years.

Aim for three hours of exercise a week. Keeping track of your exercise in a diary or on a calendar will encourage you. Stick with your new routine year round.

2. Take between 1,000 and 1,200 mg of calcium every day.

To assess your present intake, jot down everything you eat for a few days. If you already are getting the recommended amounts, go on to the next chapter; if not, consider the next few points, each of which will help give you 1,000 mg of calcium. Tables 18 and 25, on pages 92 and 104, will also help you design your own calcium-rich menu.

3. Don't forget to take 400 IU of vitamin D per day.

Vitamin D stimulates the absorption of calcium and is its essential partner. See Table 26, page 105, to learn more about this vitamin.

4. Eat at least six portions of fruits and vegetables a day.

Fruits and vegetables give you vitamins and minerals that — along with calcium — help maintain bone density. They also reduce acidity in the body and protect the calcium stored in your bones. You can't do without them. Choose foods that are richest in nutrients and vary them according to the seasons. Consider eating more of the following:

- citrus fruits like oranges, tangerines, grapefruit, limes and lemons;
- green leafy vegetables like spinach, Swiss chard, kale, collards, dandelion leaves, arugula;
- cruciferous vegetables like broccoli, cauliflower, Brussels sprouts and green or red cabbage;
- strawberries and blackberries;
- dried fruits such as figs and raisins.

See Tables 19 to 23, pages 94 to 102, for the best sources of vitamin C, vitamin K, zinc, manganese and copper. These nutrients play an important role in protecting bone density.

5. Eat boron-rich foods regularly.

Eating boron-rich foods appears to reduce the amount of calcium lost in the urine. A daily intake of 3 mg of boron is all that's needed. You can easily obtain this amount by eating enough fruits and vegetables, and a few nuts and dried fruits every day. See Table 13, page 61.

6. Moderate your protein and sodium consumption.

Two eating habits must be kept under close watch, says Dr. Robert Heaney of Creighton University: excessive intake of protein and sodium, the main causes of calcium loss in the urine.

Inuit women, who consume plenty of animal protein (at least 200 g per day), have 10 to 15% less bone mass than white women of the same age; Inuit women have a higher incidence of fractured vertebrae.

Taking in 60 g of protein a day (as suggested in Chapter 3) to maintain a good energy level is not excessive. By all means, eat a little meat, poultry or fish, but don't forget to put plant proteins such as legumes, soy and nuts on your menu, since they cause lower loss of calcium in the urine.

Limit your sodium intake to 2,000 to 3,000 mg a day. See Table 27, page 106.

> Our bones need a little care and plenty of exercise to keep them from becoming brittle.

TABLE 18

Food sources of calcium*

Food	Portion		Calcium (mg)
FRUITS AND VEGETABLES			
Beet greens, cooked	150 g	1 cup	173
Kale, cooked	130 g	1 cup	148
Dandelion greens, cooked	150 g	1 cup	147
Swiss chard, cooked	180 g	1 cup	146
Dried figs	5	5	135
Broccoli, cooked	80 g	1/2 cup	94
Orange	1	1	48
Blackberries	140 g	1 cup	46
Dried raisins	90 g	1/2 cup	43
GRAIN PRODUCTS			
Cream of Wheat, cooked	125 mL	1/2 cup	102
Bran muffin	1 medium	1 medium	57
All Bran	40 g	1/2 cup	38
Enriched white rice, cooked	180 g	1 cup	35
Bagel	1	1	29
Wholewheat bread	1 slice	1 slice	25
MEAT AND OTHER PROTEIN SOURCES			
Canned sardines with bones	90 g	3 oz.	393
Canned salmon with bones	90 g	3 oz.	183
Regular firm tofu	120 g	4 oz.	154
Canned herring with bones	90 g	3 oz.	132
Pinto beans, cooked	180 g	1 cup	130
Scallops or shrimps, cooked	90 g	3 oz.	101
White kidney beans, cooked	180 g	1 cup	98
Dried sesame seeds	8 g	1 tbs.	88
Raw oysters	90 g	3 oz.	85
Chick peas, cooked	80 g	1 cup	84

TABLE 18 cont'd

Food sources of calcium*

Food	Portion		Calcium (mg)
	MILK PRODUCTS		
Milk, calcium-enriched	250 mL	1 cup	425
Ricotta	135 g	1/2 cup	337
2%, 1% or skim milk	250 mL	1 cup	315
Plain yogurt	125 g	1/2 cup	237
Cheddar	30 g	1 oz.	216
Provolone	30 g	1 oz.	214
Skim milk powder	16 g	2 tbs.	183
Kefir	125 g	1/2 cup	175
	OTHER		
Black strap molasses	15 mL	1 tbs.	138

* Minimum calcium intake: 1,000 mg/day (age 31–50)
  (RDI 1997)   1,200 mg/day (age 51 and older)

TABLE 19
Food sources of zinc*

Food	Portion		Zinc (mg)
FRUITS AND VEGETABLES			
Green peas, cooked	80 g	1/2 cup	1.0
Spinach, cooked	90 g	1/2 cup	0.7
Collards, raw	20 g	1/2 cup	0.6
Prune juice	250 mL	1 cup	0.6
Dried figs	5	5	0.5
Avocado	1/2 medium	1/2 medium	0.4
Cantaloupe	1/2	1/2	0.4
Zucchini, cooked	90 g	1/2 cup	0.4
Banana	1 medium	1 medium	0.4
GRAIN PRODUCTS			
Dark rye flour	65 g	1/2 cup	3.6
Wheat germ	30 g	1/4 cup	2.5
Wild rice, cooked	160 g	1 cup	2.2
All Bran	20 g	1/4 cup	1.4
Brown rice, cooked	190 g	1 cup	1.2
Shredded Wheat	1 biscuit	1 biscuit	0.6
Pot barley, cooked	100 g	1/2 cup	0.6
Bagel	1	1	0.5
MEAT AND OTHER PROTEIN SOURCES			
Atlantic oysters, raw	90 g	3 oz.	82.0
Liver (calf or pork), cooked	90 g	3 oz.	6.2
Extra-lean minced beef, cooked	90 g	3 oz.	4.6
Crab, cooked	90 g	3 oz.	3.8
Turkey, cooked	90 g	3 oz.	2.8
Chick peas, cooked	180 g	1 cup	2.5
Clams, cooked	90 g	3 oz.	2.5
Pork or chicken, cooked	90 g	3 oz.	1.9
Shrimp, cooked	90 g	3 oz.	1.6

TABLE 19 cont'd
Food sources of zinc*

Food	Portion		Zinc (mg)
MEAT AND OTHER PROTEIN SOURCES CONT'D			
Red kidney beans, cooked	180 g	1 cup	1.5
Black beans, cooked	180 g	1 cup	0.9
Egg, cooked	1	1	0.6
MILK PRODUCTS			
Yogurt cheese	100 g	1/2 cup	1.9
Partially skimmed ricotta	135 g	1/2 cup	1.7
Plain yogurt	225 mL	3/4 cup	1.4
Gouda	30 g	1 oz.	1.1
2% milk	250 mL	1 cup	0.9

* Recommended nutritional intake: 9 mg/day
  (Canada 1990)

TABLE 20
Food sources of manganese*

Food	Portion		Manganese (mg)
FRUITS AND VEGETABLES			
Pineapple, fresh or juice	80 g	1/2 cup	1.3
Blackberries	70 g	1/2 cup	1.0
Spinach, cooked	90 g	1/2 cup	0.9
Chicory	50 g	1 cup	0.8
Okra, cooked	90 g	1/2 cup	0.8
Raspberries	60 g	1/2 cup	0.7
Sweet potato, puréed	125 g	1/2 cup	0.6
Kale, cooked	150 g	1 cup	0.6
Spinach, raw	60 g	1 cup	0.5
Grape juice	125 mL	1/2 cup	0.5
Green peas, cooked	80 g	1/2 cup	0.4
GRAIN PRODUCTS			
Wholewheat pasta, cooked	140 g	1 cup	2.0
Raisin Bran	55 g	1 cup	2.0
Brown rice, cooked	190 g	1 cup	1.9
Rice bran	15 mL	1 tbs.	1.5
Quick oats, cooked	240 g	1 cup	1.5
All Bran	20 g	1/4 cup	1.2
Mini-Wheats	10 biscuits	10 biscuits	0.8
Wheat bran	30 mL	2 tbs.	0.8
Millet, cooked	240 g	1 cup	0.7
Cheerios or Special K	25 g	1 cup	0.6
Pita	1	1	0.4
MEAT AND OTHER PROTEIN SOURCES			
Lima beans, cooked	180 g	1 cup	2.3
Chick peas, cooked	180 g	1 cup	1.5
White kidney beans, cooked	180 g	1 cup	1.2
Tofu, regular, firm	100 g	3.5 oz.	1.2
Lentils, cooked	180 g	1 cup	1.0

TABLE 20 cont'd

Food sources of manganese*

Food	Portion		Manganese (mg)
MEAT AND OTHER PROTEIN SOURCES CONT'D			
Pecans	18 g	2 tbs.	0.6
Liver (calf or pork), cooked	90 g	3 oz.	0.5
Pine nuts or pumpkin seeds	8 g	1 tbs.	0.4
Peanuts or sunflower seeds	16 g	2 tbs.	0.4
Almond butter	15 ml	1 tbs.	0.4
OTHER			
Tea, brewed	250 mL	1 cup	0.6

* Recommended nutritional intake: 3.5 mg/day
  (Canada 1990)

TABLE 21

Food sources of copper*

Food	Portion		Copper (mg)
FRUITS AND VEGETABLES			
Potato, baked	1	1	0.6
Vegetable juice	250 mL	1 cup	0.5
Avocado	1	1	0.5
Spinach, cooked	180 g	1 cup	0.3
Potato, boiled	1	1	0.2
Blackberries, fresh	140 g	1 cup	0.2
Kale, cooked	130 g	1 cup	0.2
Pear	1	1	0.2
Mango	170 g	1 cup	0.2
Mushrooms	35 g	1/2 cup	0.2
Pineapple	160 g	1 cup	0.2
Asparagus	90 g	1/2 cup	0.1
GRAIN PRODUCTS			
Soy flour	40 g	1/2 cup	1.6
Wild rice, cooked	160 g	1 cup	0.6
Pot barley, cooked	100 g	1/2 cup	0.2
Whole wheat pasta, cooked	140 g	1 cup	0.2
Brown rice, cooked	190 g	1 cup	0.2
Rolled oats, cooked	240 g	1 cup	0.2
Wheat germ	30 g	1/4 cup	0.1
MEAT AND OTHER PROTEIN SOURCES			
Calf liver, cooked	90 g	3 oz.	8.4
Atlantic oysters, raw	90 g	3 oz.	4.0
Beef liver, cooked	90 g	3 oz.	2.4
Clams, cooked	90 g	3 oz.	0.7
Crab, cooked	90 g	3 oz.	0.6
Chick peas, cooked	180 g	1 cup	0.6
Pork liver, cooked	90 g	3 oz.	0.5
Red kidney beans, cooked	180 g	1 cup	0.4

TABLE 21 cont'd

Food sources of copper*

Food	Portion		Copper (mg)
MEAT AND OTHER PROTEIN SOURCES CONT'D			
Regular tofu	100 g	3.5 oz.	0.4
Pumpkin seeds, roasted	18 g	2 tbs.	0.4
Lima beans, cooked	180 g	1 cup	0.4
Soy beverage	250 mL	1 cup	0.3
Mixed nuts	18 g	2 tbs.	0.2
Shrimp, cooked	90 g	3 oz.	0.2

* Recommended nutritional intake: 2 mg/day
  (Canada 1990)

TABLE 22
Food sources of vitamin C*

Food	Portion		Vitamin C (mg)
FRUITS AND VEGETABLES			
Red pepper	80 g	1/2 cup	95
Strawberries	150 g	1 cup	85
Broccoli, cooked	160 g	1 cup	82
Kiwi fruit	1	1	75
Orange	1	1	70
Cantaloupe	160 g	1 cup	68
Brussels sprouts, cooked	80 g	1/2 cup	48
Grapefruit	1	1	47
Mango	170 g	1 cup	46
Red cabbage	70 g	1 cup	40
Cauliflower	50 g	1/2 cup	36
Green cabbage	70 g	1 cup	33
Raspberries	65 g	1/2 cup	31
Potato, baked	1	1	26
Pineapple	160 g	1 cup	24
Asparagus	90 g	1/2 cup	22
Tomato	1	1	22
Cherries	170 g	1 cup	13
Cranberries	195 g	1 cup	13
Apple	1	1	8
Pear	1	1	7
Peach	1	1	6
Plum	1	1	6
SOURCES OF PROTEIN			
Lima beans, cooked	180 g	1 cup	17
Lentils, cooked	180 g	1 cup	13

* Recommended nutritional intake: 40 mg/day
  (Canada 1990)

TABLE 23
Food sources of vitamin K*

Food	Portion		Vitamin K (μg)
FRUITS AND VEGETABLES			
Spinach, raw	100 g	1 cup	298
Green kale, raw	100 g	1 cup	195
Broccoli, raw	90 g	1 cup	176
Cabbage	70 g	1 cup	104
Cauliflower	100 g	1 cup	96
Iceberg lettuce	60 g	1 cup	67
Asparagus, fresh	4 pieces	4 pieces	39
Tomato	1	1	28
Strawberries	150 g	1 cup	21
Green beans, cooked	70 g	1/2 cup	14
Carrot	1	1	9
Beets	2 medium	2 medium	8
Potato, baked	1	1	8
Orange	1	1	7
Apple	1	1	4
Mushrooms	35 g	1/2 cup	3
GRAIN PRODUCTS			
Wholewheat flour	60 g	1/2 cup	18
Wheat bran	12 g	1/4 cup	8
Wheat germ	30 g	1/4 cup	7
MEAT AND OTHER PROTEIN SOURCES			
Lentils, dried	100 g	1/2 cup	214
Soybeans, dried	100 g	1/2 cup	177
Chick peas, dried	100 g	1/2 cup	132
Beef liver, raw	90 g	3 oz.	88
Egg yolk	1 large	1 large	25
Ground beef, raw	100g	3.5 oz.	4
MILK PRODUCTS			
Skim milk	250 mL	1 cup	10

TABLE 23 cont'd
Food sources of vitamin K*

Food	Portion		Vitamin K (µg)
	OTHER		
Canola oil	15 mL	1 tbs.	115
Soy oil	15 mL	1 tbs.	68
Olive oil	15 mL	1 tbs.	8
Corn oil	15 mL	1 tbs.	7
Honey	15 mL	1 tbs.	5

* Recommended nutritional intake: 65 mg/day
  (USA 1990)

TABLE 24
Medications that affect calcium

Medication	Side effects
Antacids with an aluminum base Maalox, Mylanta, Amphojel Milk of magnesia	Increase calcium loss
Antibiotics Tetracycline, Novotetra, Erythromycine, Erythrocine, E-Mycine, Isoniazide, Isotamine	Reduce calcium absorption
Anticoagulants Heparine, Hepalen	Increase calcium loss
Hypolipidemic drugs Cholestyramine, Questran	Increase calcium loss
Diuretics Furosemide, Lasix, Uritol, Thiazide group, Thiazide	Increase calcium loss in urine Decrease calcium loss in urine
Hormonal preparations Corticosteroids, cortisone, Prednisone, Synthroid	Increase trabecular bone loss Increase bone loss

Source: Herbert and Subak-Sharpe, *Total Nutrition*, New York, St. Martin's Griffin, 1995.

TABLE 25
Suggestions for getting 1,000 mg of calcium

Food	Daily Portion	Calcium (mg)
SUGGESTION NO. 1		
Milk, calcium-enriched	250 mL (1 cup)	425
Sockeye salmon	100 g (3.5 oz.)	242
Collards, cooked	130 g (1 cup)	179
Ricotta, partly skimmed	70 g (1/4 cup)	167
Almonds	35 g (1/4 cup)	100
SUGGESTION NO. 2		
Plain yogurt	175 g (3/4 cup)	292
Cheddar cheese	30 g (1 oz.)	220
Powdered skim milk	16 g (2 tbs.)	183
White kidney beans	180 g (1 cup)	170
Orange	1	52
Wholewheat bread	2 slices	50
Broccoli, cooked	80 g (1/2 cup)	38
SUGGESTION NO. 3		
Milk	250 mL (1 cup)	315
Plain yogurt	125 g (1/2 cup)	237
Regular firm tofu	100 g (3.5 oz.)	150
Dried figs	5	135
Kale, cooked	65 g (1/2 cup)	103
Sesame seeds	40 g (1/4 cup)	52
Rice, cooked	190 g (1 cup)	24
SUGGESTION NO. 4		
Canned sardines with bones	90 g (3 oz.)	393
Soy beverage, calcium-enriched	250 mL (1 cup)	300
Swiss chard, cooked	130 g (1 cup)	146
Black strap molasses	15 mL (1 tbs.)	138
Red kidney beans, cooked	90 g (1/2 cup)	58

TABLE 26
Foods rich in vitamin D*

Food	Portion	Vitamin D (IU)
Smoked eel	30 g (1 oz.)	1,814
Pink salmon, cooked	100 g (3.5 oz.)	679
Herring, raw	30 g (1 oz.)	255
2% milk	250 mL (1 cup)	106
Canned sardines	30 g (1 oz.)	85
Egg yolk	1	27
Calf liver	90 g (3 oz.)	12
Oysters, raw	4	3

Vitamin D supplements

Product	Portion	Vitamin D (IU)
Cod liver oil	5 mL	400
Halibut liver oil (Swiss)	1 capsule	400
Vitamin D (Swiss)	1 capsule	300
Cod liver oil (Swiss)	1 capsule	100
Cod liver oil (Jamieson)	1 capsule	100
Cod liver oil (PiLeJe)	1 mL	75 to 275

Exposure to sunlight

2 to 3 times a week for 10 to 15 minutes, without sunscreen, between 8:00 a.m. and 4:00 p.m. (face, arms, hands)

* Minimum intake of vitamin D: 200 IU/day, age 20–50
  (Washington 1997)   400 IU/day, age 51–70
        600 IU/day, age 71 years and over

TABLE 27
Sodium content of selected foods

Food	Portion		Sodium (mg)
Ham and cheese sandwich	1	1	1,542
Grilled cheese sandwich	1	1	1,169
Soy sauce or tamari	15 mL	1 tbs.	1,017
Creamed chicken soup	250 mL	1 cup	870
Dill pickle	1 medium	1 medium	833
Cooked ham in slices	60 g	2 oz.	746
Canned chick peas	180 g	1 cup	718
Pizza	1 slice	1 slice	699
Smoked salmon	90 g	3 oz.	666
Smoked sausage (beef and pork)	1 (68 g)	1 (2 oz.)	642
Miso	15 mL	1 tbs.	603
Green olives	5	5	468
Parmesan cheese, grated	25 g	1/4 cup	465
Cottage cheese	135 g	1/2 cup	459
Croissant	1	1	452
Processed cheese slices	1 slice	1 slice	406
Mashed potatoes (salt and milk)	160 g	1/2 cup	318
Feta cheese	30 g	1 oz.	316
Canned anchovies in oil	2	2	300
Soy sauce, low sodium	15 mL	1 tbs.	300
Canned white tuna in water	90 g	3 oz.	300
Canned asparagus	120 g	1/2 cup	284
Barbecue sauce	30 mL	2 tbs.	258
Potato chips	20 (40 g)	20 (1 1/2 oz.)	214
Caesar salad dressing	30 mL	2 tbs.	206
Ketchup	15 mL	1 tbs.	202
Seasoned croutons	15 g	1/2 cup	200
Mustard	15 mL	1 tbs.	188

TABLE 27 cont'd

Sodium content of selected foods

Food	Portion		Sodium (mg)
Wholewheat bread	1 slice	1 slice	180
Cheddar cheese	30 g	1 oz.	176
2% milk	250 mL	1 cup	122
Butter	15 mL	1 tbs.	116
Fruit yogurt	175 g	3/4 cup	88
Chicken, cooked	90 g	3 oz.	77
Peanuts, roasted and unsalted	30 mL	2 tbs.	71
Brown rice, cooked	250 mL	1 cup	10
Eggs, boiled	1	1	62
Frozen yogurt	90 g	1/2 cup	45
Fresh spinach	100 g	1 cup	44
Canned Atlantic salmon	90 g	3 oz.	36
Carrot, raw	1	1	25
Firm tofu	120 g	4 oz.	17
Potato, baked	1	1	16
Fresh broccoli	80 g	1/2 cup	12
Tomato	1	1	11
Chick peas, cooked	180 g	1 cup	11
Shredded Wheat	2 biscuits	2 biscuits	8
Asparagus, cooked	90 g	1/2 cup	4
Kiwi fruit	1	1	4
Perrier sparkling spring water	250 mL	1 cup	2
Cream of Wheat, cooked	240 g	1 cup	2
Pasta, cooked, unsalted	140 g	1 cup	1
Apple	1	1	1
Pear	1	1	1

VIII

Treating Osteoporosis

Osteoporosis is a disease that slowly but surely erodes your body's bones. Affecting one woman in four, it normally appears in women age 70 and over. Because it afflicts twice as many women as men, osteoporosis is considered a woman's disease.

DEFINING OUR TERMS

Osteoporosis is a silent disease characterized by an *abnormally* high loss of bone tissue, as distinct from the *normal* bone loss associated with aging and menopause (discussed in chapter 7). The primary characteristic of the disease is a significant loss of bone mass and a deterioration of the internal architecture of the bones, two conditions that increase bone brittleness and the risk of fracture.

An afflicted bone is as porous as Swiss cheese with enormous holes. Small wonder then that osteoporotic bone is very fragile. A gradual weakening of the bone may be accompanied by pain, spinal cord deformation due to small, silent fractures, the loss of a few centimetres in height, and, eventually, more serious fractures. The most common are spinal fractures beginning at age 50, wrist fractures occurring before 65 and hip fractures after 80. Osteoporosis is the cause of most of the fractures that occur after menopause.

THE RISK FACTORS

As in all diseases, some women are more susceptible to osteoporosis than others. Generally speaking, women with the following profile run the greatest risk of osteoporosis.

Bone structure and body weight. Slender women have less bone mass than larger-framed women. They also have less fatty tissue covering their bones to protect them in case of a fall. A recent five-year study of 8,000 women age 65 or older reported that full-framed women suffered half as many fractures as slender women. This is why osteoporosis experts like to see women become a little plumper instead of a little thinner when they pass 50.

Race and ethnicity. Caucasian and Asian women have less bone mass and bone density than African-American women.

Heredity. A woman with a family history of bone deformation or fracture is at greater risk than one with no such history.

Inadequate intake of calcium and other nutrients. A woman who does not get the recommended quantities of essential nutrients (see Chapter 7) has less bone mass and is more susceptible to bone tissue loss.

Sedentary lifestyle. The less demand you put on your skeleton, the less bone density and bone strength you maintain. A report published by the Canadian Institute for Fitness and Lifestyle Research shows that two-thirds of Canadian men and women get too little exercise and become even less active with age.

Smoking. Tobacco and, more specifically, nicotine, decrease calcium use and diminish estrogen circulation. Recently, the *British Medical Journal* published a summary of some 50 bone density studies done on women smokers and non-smokers. The authors concluded that, before menopause, all groups showed comparable bone density and fracture risk. But after menopause, compared with the non-smokers, the smokers lost 2% more of their bone density every 10 years, and their fracture risk was 17% greater at age 60, 41% greater at age 70 and 71% greater at age 80. The authors also concluded that one in eight fractures occurring in women who smoke could be attributed to nicotine.

Other predisposing factors

Calcium is so vital to bone health that anything that hampers its absorption or increases its elimination may worsen the situation.

- Conditions such as chronic diarrhea do not allow adequate calcium absorption.
- Medications like corticosteroids, anticonvulsants, strong doses of thyroid extracts, and aluminum-based antacids hamper calcium absorption (see Table 24, page 103).
- Your emotional state also plays a role. Stress, anxiety, grief and boredom reduce bowel absorption of calcium. Dr. David Michelson noted that women in depression had lower bone density than non-depressed women of the same age and height.

Detecting osteoporosis

Osteoporosis works as insidiously as cholesterol. You will feel no pain before either a fracture or heart attack. But today's preventive medicine can still detect the problem before it's too late.

Blood tests won't give you all the information you need. A normal calcium blood level can't tell you whether you have the disease, but other tests can detect significant bone calcium losses.

Simple bone X-rays aren't reliable either; they are not sensitive enough to detect small losses of bone. By the time an X-ray can detect it, bone loss is already significant.

Heel ultrasound is a new, inexpensive procedure that measures the bone density of the heel by immersing it in a basin of warm water through which high-frequency sounds are transmitted. The test makes it possible to assess heel bone density and solidity, but unlike bone densitometry, it doesn't identify the degree of osteoporosis. Heel ultrasound can be useful as an initial diagnostic tool.

Bone densitometry is a test that uses low doses of radiation to measure bone mass; it can predict the risk of fracture. At present, Dual Energy X-ray Absorptiometry (DEXA) is the most widely used and most accurate bone densitometry technique; it evaluates the bone density of the spinal column and/or the hips, and it can also be used for other measurements.

Once the test is completed, your bones are compared with those of a young 35- to 40-year-old adult with optimal bone mass. Although you normally lose bone mass as you grow older, the comparison indicates whether your losses are acceptable for your age or are more rapid than expected. The World Health Organization has established a standard for bone loss measurement, which is used throughout the world to detect osteoporosis.

Normal bone mass has a density of about 1 g/cm^2. Any deviation from this norm is a sign of abnormality and is expressed as Standard Deviation (SD).

- If your bone mass is about normal — between (–1) and (+1) — your risk of fracture is very low, and you do not have osteoporosis.
- If your results deviate a bit from the norm — between (–1) and (–2.5) — your bone mass has been reduced, and your risk of fracture is slightly increased. You do not have osteoporosis, but you do have *osteopenia*.
- If your score is lower than –2.5, you have osteoporosis, and your risk of fracture is higher.

SLOWING DOWN OSTEOPOROSIS

Don't feel discouraged if the bone density test shows that you are osteopenic or osteoporotic, because you can still slow the progress of the disease, improve your bone mass and reduce your risk of fracture. It's never too late to take action! Treatments tested on elderly women at risk have raised hopes that it is possible to significantly lower the incidence of fractures.

I suggest you follow an action plan that includes nutritional adjustments, dietary supplements if necessary, and substantially increased physical activity. I also recommend that you stop smoking.

Some biophosphate-based medications such as etidronate (Didronel), etidronate and calcium (Didrocal) and alendronate (Fosamax) or the new selective estrogen receptor modulators such as raloxifene (Evista) may be useful. These non-hormonal medications have been shown to be as effective as hormone replacement therapy to minimize bone loss.

PATHWAYS TO A SOLUTION
1. Take between 1,200 and 1,500 mg of calcium per day.
An adequate daily calcium supplement can slow losses by 30 to 50% — nothing to be sneezed at.

If you are already getting an abundant supply of milk products, check your calcium intake and adjust your milk consumption accordingly. If you're not a milk drinker, or you almost never eat yogurt or cheese, consider the other suggestions about calcium-rich foods and boost your menu with green leafy vegetables, broccoli, soy beverages, etc. If, for whatever reason, you can't manage to eat calcium-rich foods regularly, take a calcium supplement and take it at the right time (see Tables 28 and 29, pages 117 and 118).

You may have heard that calcium intake isn't all that important, and that some women are better off using fewer milk products. Don't believe it. It is true, for instance, that compared with Canadian women, Chinese women consume less calcium and still have a lower incidence of osteoporosis. But bear in mind that Chinese women are smaller, have a smaller bone mass and are much more physically active than Canadian women, who are rather sedentary. And a study conducted in five regions in China showed that elderly women who had a higher consumption of milk products had even greater bone density.

You should increase your calcium intake even if you are taking hormones, because estrogen alone is not the answer. A summary of some 20 studies on the issue concluded that bone mass is regenerated more effectively when hormone replacement therapy is combined with a calcium intake of at least 1,200 mg a day. Spine bone mass increased by 3.3% a year when a good dose of calcium was added, compared with 1.3% when estrogen alone was used. Hipbone mass was increased by 2.4% per year, compared with 0.9% without additional calcium.

2. Don't forget to take 800 units a day of vitamin D.

Vitamin D is an indispensable partner: it stimulates calcium absorption and helps maintain the integrity of the bone structure. A study involving 400 elderly people showed that a vitamin D supplement given together with a calcium supplement could, over a three-year period, cut by half the incidence of non-vertebral fractures. Even so, many women suffer from a vitamin D deficiency. In the summer of 1997, a committee of Canadian and American experts at the National Academy of Sciences raised the recommended daily intake to remedy this widespread deficiency. The committee now recommends that women take:

200 IU per day between ages 19 and 50;
400 IU per day between ages 51 and 70;
600 IU per day after age 71.

Vitamin D is not like the other vitamins: it is produced by the sun's rays, which cause the spontaneous conversion of a pre-vitamin substance under the skin. This substance becomes an active vitamin on exposure to sunlight.

Don't always count on the rays of the sun alone, though, for your vitamin D requirements; they can play tricks on you. In equatorial regions, there is no shortage of sunlight for sure, but in regions north of the 40th parallel (New York, Montreal, Paris, London and Beijing), there is not enough sunlight from October to March to allow vitamin D to be activated. Even mid-summer sun is not a reliable source as it cannot penetrate sunscreens or darker skins.

The few foods that contain vitamin D are cod liver oil, halibut oil, herring, mackerel, sardines, salmon, egg yolk and butter. By law, the vitamin must be added to the milk you buy, including skim, powder, concentrated and whole milk. One glass provides about 100 IU. Vitamin D is also added to goat's milk and some soy beverages.

Vitamin D is particularly important when calcium intake is not very high, which is the case for too many women. So don't risk a vitamin D deficiency, and don't count on the sun. If you have osteoporosis, take 800 IU of vitamin D a day. To get that much vitamin D, you need a supplement (see Table 26, page 105).

3. Step up your zinc, copper and manganese intake.

Calcium has a powerful effect on bone health, but it's no panacea. It must work in tandem with vitamin D, and it is even more effective when your intake of zinc, copper and manganese is increased.

A few years ago, a study of menopausal women in California verified the effect of calcium combined with the other minerals. The researchers monitored 60 women who had been menopausal for at least six years. The participants were given various supplements: some took a placebo, others received only 1,000 mg of calcium, and still others took an additional supplement of 15 mg of zinc, 5 mg of manganese and 2.5 mg of copper. None of them took hormones. The study was double blind; that is, neither the researchers nor the women knew what supplements, if any, the subjects were receiving. The bone density of the spinal column was measured at the beginning of the study, and again after two years. The researchers noted that women who had taken calcium alone or minerals alone had less bone density loss than women who had taken a placebo. In addition, researchers noted a significant increase in bone density among the women who had taken both supplements.

You can fortify your menu with foods that are good sources of zinc, manganese and copper (see Tables 19, 20 and 21, pages 94 to 99). You can also purchase multivitamins and minerals that contain 15 mg of zinc, 5 mg of manganese and 2.5 mg of copper.

4. Cut your calcium losses.

Reduce your sodium consumption. As you have seen, it isn't easy to get calcium in sufficient quantities, and calcium isn't easy to absorb or retain. We lose it in stool, urine and sweat, but there are only a few ways to minimize the losses. One of them is to eat less salt.

With every 100 mg of sodium in your food, you lose 1 mg of calcium in your urine. The more you eat foods rich in sodium, the more calcium you lose. If you crave fast food, frozen food and restaurant meals, if you love munching on crackers and chips, or if you add salt to your food instead of herbs or spices, your high sodium intake can trigger a major calcium loss, despite your best efforts to get the right amount.

To retain as much calcium as possible, limit your sodium consumption to between 2,000 and 3,000 mg a day. Avoid foods rich in sodium, like cold meats, prepared soups, bouillon bases, soy sauces, sodium glutamate, garlic or onion salts, cheese spreads and canned foods (see Table 27, page 106). Season with herbs, spices, lemon juice, balsamic vinegar, garlic and/or onions.

Eat less animal protein. Eating too much animal protein (meat, chicken and fish) weakens the bone mass by increasing calcium losses in the urine. Some Japanese researchers contend that consuming plant proteins like soy and legumes does not appear to cause the same losses. The difference between calcium losses arising from a meat-based menu and those arising from a vegetarian menu has been estimated at 50 mg per day.

Still, if your vegetarian menu is too strict, doesn't contain enough proteins and doesn't allow you to maintain a healthy body weight, it can also reduce your bone density. A study of 258 vegetarian Buddhists in Taiwan showed that extreme thinness and low protein intakes were associated with osteopenia and substantially increased the risk of osteoporosis.

Moderate protein consumption consists of about 60 g/day (see Table 30, page 120). If you distribute protein-rich foods throughout your menu in order to have enough at each meal, and if you alternate between animal proteins and plant proteins, you'll have plenty of energy, and you'll cut your calcium losses in the bargain.

You can eat moderately and enjoy it, too!

5. Increase your physical activity

Strengthen your muscles; take a 30-minute walk every day. Exercise can work miracles. After a year of exercise twice a week, menopausal women increased their bone mass by 1% compared with sedentary women, who saw it decrease by 2.5%. The women who exercised also significantly increased their muscle mass and strength.

> By simply taking a daily walk, you can also reduce the risk of fracture. So, no more excuses!

TABLE 28
Which calcium supplement is for you?

Any calcium supplement can help you reach your goal of
1,200 to 1,500 mg of calcium a day.

Carbonate-based supplements are more concentrated; they
provide more calcium in each tablet and must be taken with food, during
a snack or meal, for better absorption. They are reasonably priced.

Citrate-based or citrate/malate-based supplements are more
easily absorbed. They don't cause digestive problems and can be
taken at any time of the day. They are more expensive than
carbonate-based supplements.

Other forms of calcium like **fumarate, glucomate** and
succinate have no particular qualities, but they are often
integrated into carbonates or citrates.

Chelate calcium is coated with an amino acid compound, which
guards against the negative action of fibres like phytates in cereals and
oxalates in spinach or in rhubarb. Calcium absorption is also increased
by 5 to 10%, but calcium chelate is very expensive.

Some supplements contain **bone meal** or **dolomite**, two other
sources of calcium that seem easily absorbed.

Note the amount of **elemental calcium** on the label;
it indicates the amount of calcium retained. Ask your pharmacist
for the information if it isn't given on the label.

You can absorb calcium more easily if you divide it into small
doses taken one at a time. If you need a supplement of 1,000 mg per day,
spread the doses out, taking, for example, 500 mg in the morning and
500 mg in the evening or 300 mg after each meal.

If you don't drink milk and don't take multivitamins and
minerals, look for a calcium supplement that contains vitamin D.
If the dose of vitamin D doesn't suit you, find a
vitamin D supplement with a fish-oil base.

If you have kidney stones, get your calcium in food, not in supplements. Dietary calcium inhibits kidney stone formation from oxalates.
Drink plenty of water — about two litres (eight cups) a day.

TABLE 29
Calcium supplements

	Elemental calcium (mg)
Calcium carbonate	
Calcrate 600 (Whitehall Robbins)	600
Calcite 500	500
Calsan (Sandoz)	500
Os-Cal 500	500
Tums, liquid	400/5 mL
Tums, tablets, extra strength	300
Tums, tablets, regular strength	200
Cal-K (Somapharm)	150
Calcium carbonate with vitamin D	
Calcrate 600 + D	600
Calcium D 500 (Laboratoires Trianon)	500
Cal-500-D (Prodoc)	500
Sisu: calcium/magnesium, vitamin D	480/30 mL
Adrien Gagnon: calcium/magnesium, vitamin D and zinc	350
Swiscal: calcium/magnesium, vitamin D, iron and zinc	333
Menocal: calcium/magnesium, vitamins B12 and D, iron and zinc	333
Swiscal: calcium/magnesium, vitamins B12 and D, and zinc	200
Calcium citrate	
Calcium Citrate (Swiss)	350
Citracal	200
Cal-Citrus	200
Natural Factors Citrate plus: calcium/magnesium, vitamin D, manganese, potassium and zinc	125

TABLE 29 cont'd
Calcium supplements

	Elemental calcium (mg)
Calcium citrate with vitamin D	
Natural Factors Citrate plus D: calcium/ magnesium, vitamin D, manganese, potassium and zinc	315
Citrate Cal-Mag (Swiss): calcium/magnesium, vitamin D and zinc	300
Citracal + vitamin D	250
Other supplements	
Gramcal Sandoz	1,000
Calcium-Sandoz, strong (effervescent tablets)	500
Liquicks: calcium/magnesium, vitamin D and zinc	400/30 mL
Opti-Cal/Mag: calcium/magnesium, vitamin D and zinc	350
Calais, sparkling drink (Mead Johnson)	300/350 mL
Floradix Liquid: calcium/magnesium, vitamin D and zinc	155/30 mL
Calcium Sandoz	110/5 mL
Quest Cal-Mag: calcium/magnesium and vitamin D	100

TABLE 30
Sample Meals that Include Protein*

Meal	Food	Proteins (g)
	Menu containing over 60 g of protein	
Breakfast	Orange juice	
	Creamed **Tofu** with Fruit	12
Snack	Small glass of **milk**	4
Lunch	Green bean and yellow bell pepper salad	
	Turkey and cranberry pita	15
	Kiwi fruit	
Snack	**Yogurt**	7
Supper	Endive	
	Wholewheat spaghetti	8
	Tomato sauce with **lentils** and grated	13
	Parmesan	
	Orange slices	
	Menu containing over 100 g of protein	
Breakfast	Orange juice	
	2 eggs	13
	Wholewheat toast and **peanut butter**	10
Snack	Apple and **cheese**	8
Lunch	Green bean and yellow bell pepper salad	
	Turkey and cranberry pita	15
	Yogurt and kiwi fruit	8
Supper	**Steak** with three peppers	45
	Potato	
	Green salad	
	Vanilla **ice cream**	5

* Foods indicated in boldface are rich in protein.

IX

Preventing Breast Cancer

There is no *direct* link between breast cancer and menopause, since 20% of all cases are diagnosed in women before age 40. Most cases do, however, occur in women 55 or older. The incidence of breast cancer may be increasing, but the chances of survival are greater than ever before. Three out of four women get a clean bill of health five years after they begin treatment.

At the time of writing, I am working as a volunteer dietitian with a team of 24 dragon boat rowers, all of whom are breast cancer survivors. They've completed their treatment — and decided to put their trust in life and in the strength of their bodies. During the summers of 1998 and 1999, they competed in at least seven important races, so they had to improve their diet to meet the added demands of training. How I admire their energy and courage! Even though they are past the prevention stage, I dedicate this chapter to them.

Studies increasingly show that protective foods can become healing foods.

GOOD NUTRITION FOR ADDED PROTECTION

In 1997, an expert committee of the American Institute for Cancer Research (AICR) stated that women could reduce the incidence of breast cancer by 30 to 50% by following a better diet and getting more exercise.

It's a fact: breast cancer is much more widespread in the industrialized countries, where nutrition is inadequate and physical activity deficient. Japan is the exception to the rule: the breast cancer rate for Japanese women is four times lower than that for American women. Researchers studying this peculiarity focused on soy. They noted that Japanese women who regularly consume soy exhibit a lower incidence of breast cancer than those who don't. But when Japanese women move to the United States and change their eating habits, their daughters suffer as much from the disease as other American women of the same generation.

Another surprising fact: while the link between excess dietary fat and breast cancer has long been discussed, the focus has now shifted to the kind of fat consumed, rather than the quantity. For example, Inuit women who consume a great deal of omega type-3 fats (good fats) and Mediterranean women who consume plenty of olive oil (another good fat) have a lower incidence of breast cancer than North American women who consume less fat overall but a higher proportion of hydrogenated and saturated fats.

DOES DIET AFFECT HORMONE LEVELS?

A number of studies on breast cancer in menopausal women have linked high blood estrogen and testosterone levels with the onset of the disease. Other researchers have hypothesized that a change in nutrition might reduce the hormone level in the bloodstream and therefore might also reduce breast cancer risk. We now know some of the factors that increase the hormone level in the blood.

Alcohol consumption raises hormonal concentration in the blood and increases the risk of breast cancer. The latest risk assessment published in the *Journal of the American Medical Association* in February 1998 reviewed six major studies involving 322,000 women, carried out in Canada, the United States, Sweden and Holland. The authors concluded that with every additional 10 g of alcohol per day, the risk increased by 9%. Alcohol consumption is as significant a risk factor as family history. Several other studies have reached similar conclusions (see Table 31, page 128).

Post-menopausal obesity also has a significant impact on the hormone level; the more fatty tissue a woman has, the more *androstendione* is converted into estrogen. The more estrogen in the bloodstream, the more vulnerable breast tissue becomes to cancer.

> *Androstendione* is the hormone produced by the suprarenal glands located just above the kidneys. After menopause, when the ovaries no longer produce estrogen, androstendione is converted into estrogen in the fatty tissue. The plumper a woman is, the more estrogen is circulating in her blood. Her bones will benefit from the extra estrogen, but she becomes more vulnerable to breast cancer.

Conversely, some foods appear to reduce the hormone level in the bloodstream. To determine the impact of nutrition on hormones, a team of Italian scientists recruited 104 menopausal women in Milan who weren't taking hormones and who had high testosterone levels; these women were considered at risk for breast cancer. Half of them made no change in their diet. The other half made significant changes: they increased their daily intake of foods rich in phytoestrogens (soy, legumes and flaxseed), foods rich in fibres (whole grains and legumes), foods rich in omega-3 fats (fish, walnuts and green leafy vegetables), cruciferous vegetables, and berries. They also ate less meat, cheese and refined sugar. After six months, the women who had modified their diet saw their testosterone level drop by 18% and their Sex Hormone Binding Globulin Level (SHBG) rise by 23%.

> SHBG (sex hormone binding globulin) is a protein that circulates in the blood. It adheres to testosterone and, to a lesser extent, to estrogen. Increased SHBG in the blood reduces the concentration of free hormones and lowers the risk of breast cancer.
>
> For example, in comparison with British women, Japanese women have more SHBG and a lower incidence of breast cancer.

The food we eat has such a marked effect on blood hormone levels that the authors of the Italian study concluded that this diet could reduce the incidence of breast cancer by 25 to 30%.

Several other studies have examined the effect of some foods on the hormone level in the bloodstream.

We now know, for instance, that a dose of 10 g (1/4 cup) of wheat bran per day can lower blood estrogen levels. Other fibre-rich foods can have the same effect.

Some fascinating research has also focused on foods rich in **isoflavones, lignans, carotenoids, indoles** and **flavonoids**. The studies first identified these substances, then demonstrated their anticarcinogenic action mechanisms.

Isoflavones are the phytoestrogens found in soy (see Table 11, page 59). These estrogen-like substances can compete with our own estrogen, increase the production of SBGH and reduce the circulation of estrogen in the blood. They act much like an antiestrogen and have been compared to Tamoxifen, a well-known antiestrogenic medication. They cannot replace such medication but can act in a similar fashion. The low breast cancer rate among Japanese women who live in Japan and regularly consume soy is the most striking example of the protective effect of isoflavones.

Lignans are the phytoestrogens present in flaxseed and whole grain products. Like soy, they limit the production and circulation of estrogen and thus have an anticarcinogenic effect. But don't count on flaxseed oil, which, unlike flaxseed itself, contains little or no lignans.

Carotenoids are a large group of antioxidant substances. Except for the properties of beta-carotene, they were unknown 10 years ago. They are found in darker coloured fruits and vegetables such as carrots, sweet potatoes, tomatoes, spinach, broccoli, cantaloupe and apricots, and are now considered anticarcinogenic agents. A study conducted in five American states and involving 13,000 women measured the effect of vegetables rich in carotenoids and concluded that two servings of carrots and/or spinach a week lowered the breast cancer risk by 40%.

Indoles, found in the cruciferous family (broccoli, cauliflower, and Brussels sprouts, as well as green and red cabbages), can also reduce the risk of breast cancer by converting estrogen into antiestrogenic by-products.

Flavonoids, present in oranges, grapefruit, lemons, limes, onions and some cabbages, are also considered anticarcinogenic agents.

As you can see, many anticarcinogens can be found in vibrantly coloured vegetables, whole grains and soy, as well as in garlic, ginger, liquorice, celery, coriander, parsley and many other foods. Despite the fact that vitamins E and C are well known for their antioxidant properties, there is no evidence that taking them in the form of supplements can provide the same protection as regular consumption of these beneficial foods.

PATHWAYS TO PREVENTION

Several flavourful foods can play an active role in preventing breast cancer. Some of them may not yet be part of your regular diet, but they are well worth seeking out — and eating regularly.

1. Add foods rich in phytoestrogens to your daily menu.

Remember, there are two kinds of phytoestrogens: isoflavones and lignans.

Among the richest sources of isoflavones are soy flour, soy protein isolate, roasted or cooked soybeans, tofu, soy beverages, powdered soy protein, tempeh and foods containing soy (see Tables 10, 11 and 12, pages 56 to 60). And don't forget that soy contains other anticarcinogens identified in numerous studies. Don't rely on soy sauce, tamari or soy oil, however: they don't contain the substances you're looking for.

Flaxseed is one of best sources of lignans. Trailing far behind are whole grains and their cereal by-products, some vegetables and berries.

To get the full benefit of their protective action, you should include one or two servings of foods rich in soy and 10 to 15 mL (2 tsp. to 1 tbs.) of ground flaxseed in your daily diet.

Consult the recipes on pages 47 to 49 for ways to prepare or incorporate soy into the food you eat. Buy your flaxseed in bulk (normally available at the natural food store), store in the refrigerator, and use a small coffee grinder to grind to a powder. Mix 10 to 15 mL (2 tsp. to 1 tbs.) of the powder with your breakfast cereal, with yogurt or with Creamed Tofu and Fruit, or even in stewed fruit.

2. Increase your intake of cruciferous or darker coloured vegetables.

Become a part-time food colourist — put the darkest green and the brightest orange on your table every day:

- Start your meal with a glass of tomato juice, if you don't have any brightly coloured vegetables.
- Munch on baby carrots while you prepare your meal.
- Make crunchy coleslaw more often, and throw in apples and walnuts.
- Add spinach or arugula leaves to your green salads, or slip a leaf of spinach into your sandwich.
- Discover new greens like Swiss chard, collards, kale and dandelion leaves, all of which are rich in vitamins; steam them and sprinkle them with lemon juice and a few drops of olive oil.
- Prepare attractive mixed vegetables with broccoli, cubed sweet potatoes, green peas and a few carrots; cook them in the microwave

and season them with pesto. As tasty as it is colourful!

- The more vegetables you eat, the greater the health dividends. And many fruits like cantaloupe and citrus fruits are just as good.

3. Keep fat in your diet — in moderation.

It's wise to limit your total fat intake in order to maintain a healthy body weight and ensure a balanced menu, but you can still consume the omega-3 fats found in fish, seafood, algae and flaxseed.

You can also use olive oil in small quantities without increasing your risk. And experts recommend that you cut back on your intake of meat, butter and cheese, which are major sources of saturated animal fat. If you can completely avoid hydrogenated fats (see Table 1, page 8), so much the better.

4. Increase your intake of legumes and whole grains.

If you eat plenty of legumes, you'll get high-quality proteins, and you can dispense with some of your meat-based meals. Chick peas, lentils and kidney beans also provide you with fibre, which can lower the estrogen level in the bloodstream and increase the amount of SHBG, thus reducing breast cancer risk.

Whole grains and their by-products are also effective because of their lignan and fibre content. Cereal brans and germs contain the largest amount of active substances; white bread, white rice and other refined products have lost much of their nutritive value.

5. Cut your alcohol intake to a minimum.

Experts say that it's acceptable to drink a glass of wine, beer or other alcohol a day. But it's not compulsory, of course! (See Table 31, page 128.)

> Rediscover fruits, vegetables and whole grains; add soy and flaxseed to your diet and you'll strengthen your resistance to breast cancer.

TABLE 31
Alcohol content in selected alcoholic beverages

Beverage	Quantity	Alcohol (g)
BEER		
Ordinary	360 mL (12 oz.)	13
Light	360 mL (12 oz.)	10
Extra-light	360 mL (12 oz.)	8
0.5%	360 mL (12 oz.)	2
SPIRITS AND OTHERS		
Martini	90 mL (3 oz.)	19
Gin, rum, vodka and whisky	45 mL (1.5 oz.)	15
Brandy and cognac	30 mL (1 oz.)	11
WINE		
Vermouth, dry	90 mL (3 oz.)	13
Red wine	120 mL (4 oz.)	12
Vermouth, sweet	90 mL (3 oz.)	12
White wine, dry	120 mL (4 oz.)	11
Sherry	60 mL (2 oz.)	9
Port	60 mL (2 oz.)	7

Source: H. A. Guthrie and M. F. Picciano, *Human Nutrition*. St. Louis: Mosby, 1995.

X

The Winning Formula for Menopause

1. An appetizing menu
2. Three *good* protein-rich meals a day, with snacks if needed
3. Soy, in various forms, and flaxseed, *every day*
4. Plenty of fresh fruits and vegetables *every day*
5. Good fats — olive or canola oil — for salads and cooking. On the menu: fatty fish, nuts and avocados *in moderate quantities*
6. Low-fat milk products, or other good sources of calcium and vitamin D, *every day*
7. Green leafy vegetables, legumes, whole grains and other mineral-rich foods *regularly*
8. Daily physical activity: at least a 30-minute walk *every day*
9. Appropriate supplements when necessary

By now, your head is swimming with information. This book has given you all the nutritional advice you need to help you solve specific problems and to prevent disease in the future. Now you'd like to know what to eat to help you through menopause as comfortably as possible — and into a healthy, enjoyable old age. Here then is the winning formula that will see you through this period of hormonal transition.

These recommendations do not replace well-known nutritional guidelines. Quite the opposite, they complement those guidelines. They take into account your nutritional deficiencies, reorient your food choices and lead you toward an enjoyable and healthy daily routine.

Read each of the following sections carefully. Make gradual changes in your menu, and discover new food delights. You'll be the winner.

REDISCOVER THE JOY OF EATING

Many women still believe that rich fried food, sweets and chocolate are synonymous with pleasure or fun food. It's time to dispel the confusion between gluttony and good eating. Make a list of your most memorable meals and your favourite dishes; you'll be surprised at the variety of interesting foods that come to mind.

When I drew up my own list a few years ago, I discovered that my eating pleasure wasn't limited to the taste of the food. It began with the little treasures I unearthed at the market: fresh, crunchy green vegetables; ripe, tasty fruit, garden-fresh herbs; fish that smell of the sea; wholegrain bread hot from the oven. Whenever I leaf through my recipe books, my mouth waters. At the dinner table, fresh, tasty, well-prepared food is always a source of delight, but the table setting, the atmosphere and the good company give the evening that extra sparkle. The joy of eating is somewhat like a gift I offer myself by buying beautiful and nutritious foods, by preparing and serving them with tender loving care. It's a ritual I observe as often as I possibly can.

Think about it; you'll see that the joy of eating doesn't necessarily mean wolfing down potato chips, fries or chocolate cake. It has to do with many little things, like buying the food and choosing the recipe. It also has to do with the décor, company, atmosphere, tablecloth, dishes and your mood. Pay attention to these factors — tangible and intangible — and you can give your meals that added glow that translates into pure pleasure.

Rediscover the exquisite taste of food in all its freshness; nothing can be easier — or better for your eating pleasure:

- Squeeze a few oranges that have been left overnight at room temperature; savour this sweet, aromatic juice at breakfast.
- Buy fillets of fresh fish rather than the frozen variety; cook them until they are no longer transparent; they will melt in your mouth.
- Use fresh herbs like chives, thyme and basil in your recipes, tripling the called-for amount of dried herbs; taste the difference.
- Use extra-virgin olive oil and shine a little Mediterranean sunlight on your salads or leafy green vegetables.

As the famous French author Jean-François Revel writes, knowing how to mix and match good foods and their flavours is as important as evaluating their nutritional value.

Take the time to savour your food; no one will scold you, and it doesn't cost a thing!

If you no longer enjoy cooking:

- Simplify your recipes, but always look for the freshest food.
- Get inspiration from new cookbooks or magazines; look for dishes with ingredients that are easy to find, and follow simple preparation methods.
- Find a restaurant or caterer that will prepare dishes with plenty of proteins, good fats, lots of raw and barely cooked vegetables.
- Treat yourself to the joy of dining in pleasant surroundings with good company to the sound of beautiful music.

NEVER SKIP A MEAL

When you eat at least three meals a day, you're never famished or overcome by sudden food cravings. There's no need for after-supper snacks. You'll experience a kind of internal peace. At the same time, you'll stimulate your metabolic rate instead of burdening your system, which has already been slowed down by menopause. You can even stop gaining weight, instead of adding kilos in spite of yourself. You'll have more energy, and you'll absorb many of the key nutrients, such as calcium, much more easily.

Don't forget that a *good* meal contains an adequate supply of proteins (at least 15 g), two generous portions of raw or cooked vegetables, a fresh fruit and a wholewheat cereal product.

Never underestimate the importance of proteins in getting your day off to a good start at breakfast. A liquid breakfast can do the job.

- In a blender put 200 mL (3/4 cup) of milk and 60 g (2 oz.) of silken tofu; add 125 g (4 oz.) of fresh or frozen unsweetened strawberries and a drop of honey; blend until smooth. Pour and enjoy.

If you want your metabolic rate to do its work efficiently, don't eat too many rich foods at the same meal. It's better to eat more often than to eat too much at one time. If you feel hungry between meals, take time out for a healthy snack.

If you don't feel hungry in the morning, but you're ravenous by evening, that's not a good excuse. Try to eat a *good* meal a few mornings in a row and you'll see that your appetite will quickly adjust to your new schedule. You'll have the feeling you're eating more, but you'll really be eating better.

If you just don't have time to eat, change your schedule, and think of your meals as compulsory food breaks. There's no law against it.

MAKE PHYTOESTROGENS A PART OF YOUR DAILY DIET

Recent studies on cardiovascular disease, breast cancer and menopause-related diseases have clearly shown that phytoestrogen-rich foods can provide substantial short- and long-term health benefits for women.

If you are not suffering from a specific problem, make soy and flaxseed a regular part of your diet. But if you have a cholesterol problem, hot flashes or a family history of breast cancer, be a little stricter with yourself: take approximately 75 mg of isoflavones (found in soy) and a tablespoon of ground flaxseed every day. There's no other way to enjoy the known benefits of phytoestrogens.

- Use regular or silken tofu to make mousses, creams or sauces; avoid low-fat tofu — it's lost part of its phytoestrogens.
- Drink soy beverages enriched with calcium and vitamin D.
- If you can't consume enough tofu or soy beverage, eat other products containing soy, or complement your menu with soy protein isolate (see Table 8, page 51). There are plenty of products to choose from.
- Eat 15 mL (1 tbs.) of ground flaxseed every day. Flaxseed is an excellent source of lignans, which are phytoestrogens too. Not only do they have a beneficial effect on cardiovascular health and cancer prevention, but they also nourish the skin since they are rich in omega-3 fatty acids.
- Use a mortar or small coffee grinder to grind the flaxseed to a powder; it is easier to digest in this form. Mix the powder with stewed fruit or with Creamed Tofu with Fruit, yogurt or a bowl of cereal.

Eat more fruits and vegetables,
at every meal

Whether you want to maintain a healthy weight, fight constipation or hypertension, prevent cancer, or guard against excess acidity in the body, research shows that fruits and vegetables provide excellent protection. But despite all the advantages they offer — their rich content of vitamins, minerals, fibre and bioactive substances — we tend to overlook them in our diet.

- Assess your diet; if you are eating eight to 10 portions of fruits and vegetables per day, you're already following a winning formula. If not, you have some catching up to do.
- Consult Tables 32 and 33 on pages 142 and 143. You'll see that these winning foods are deeply coloured.
- Be daring; seek out less well-known fruits and vegetables. Stop off at the fruit store or the market; ask the staff for advice, if necessary. Choose the freshest fruit because freshness is a guarantee of nutritional value.
- Go green. Eat more leafy green vegetables like collards, bok choy, kale or Swiss chard; steam them and sprinkle them with lemon juice and a few drops of olive oil.
- Sample the more exotic fruits like mangoes, papayas, persimmons or passion fruit. They're so aromatic that one mouthful transports you to faraway places. Try half a papaya with lime juice, or a quarter cantaloupe with a few ripe strawberries or blackberries in season. Don't forget watermelon; it ranks high among the most nourishing fruits.
- If generous helpings of raw vegetables cause you gastrointestinal distress, reduce your intake, and use a juicer to make homemade juices, prepare salads from finely grated vegetables, which are easier to digest, or steam them just enough to tenderize the fibres.
- If you can't tolerate uncooked fruit, you can make smooth purées in the blender and mix them with fruit juice or yogurt. Poach the fruit in fruit juice, or cook in the microwave for a few minutes, just long enough to tenderize.

If you hesitate before eating fruit at the end of a meal, sit back and read what follows.

Digestive enzymes are much more efficient than some advocates of food combinations believe. These enzymes have the power to quickly act on the fruits you eat at any time during the meal. There is no better dessert than fresh fruit. If you want to ease your digestive problems, beware of fried foods. They remain in your stomach a long time; cooked fat takes much longer to digest, even if you eat it at the beginning of your meal.

When you eat more fruits and vegetables, you can't go wrong. Not only do they provide you with protective nutrients, they add colour and flavour to your meals.

KEEP GOOD FATS IN YOUR DIET

The fat debate has generated more heat than light. Many people have declared total war on fat. But many recent studies point to the beneficial effects of a moderate intake of monounsaturated or omega-3 fats (good fats). Monounsaturated fats have proven cardiovascular benefits, while omega-3 fats are transformed into extremely beneficial anti-inflammatory substances.

Eating a moderate amount of good fats is better for your arteries and your immune system than consuming fat-free foods or foods that contain fake fats.

Among the best sources of monounsaturated fats are extra-virgin olive oil, canola and hazelnut oils, as well as nuts, avocados and olives. Use the oils, rather than any other fatty substances, in cooking and for salad dressings. But don't use these oils for frying, because they will lose their nutritional value and slow down digestion.

When you feel hungry, treat yourself to some almonds, walnuts and hazelnuts, all of which supply good fat. Cookies, crackers and potato chips contain bad fat.

Among the best sources of omega-3 fats are fish such as salmon, mackerel, herring, trout and sardines. Walnuts, flaxseed and soy also contain these fats. Don't hesitate to eat fish in variety several times a week. Use flaxseed and soy as suggested above.

USE LOW-FAT MILK PRODUCTS OR FIND VALID SUBSTITUTES

Despite recent anti-milk campaigns, it's in your best interest to keep low-fat milk products on your daily menu; they are the easiest sources of calcium to consume. They also provide substantial amounts of protein and B vitamins. Though they are not irreplaceable and don't offer guaranteed protection against osteoporosis, they are healthful, nutritious foods.

Both whole and skim milk contain over 300 mg of calcium per 250 mL (1 cup). The new milks fortified with milk derivatives contain 425 mg per 250 mL (1 cup). In both cases, vitamin D, which promotes calcium absorption, is added.

Both low-fat and regular yogurts supply nearly 300 mg of calcium per 175 g (6 oz). Fruit yogurts contain more sugar, and therefore less calcium. Kefir, rich in active bacterial agents, contains 350 mg per 250 mL (1 cup), and some fresh aromatic cheeses provide 200 mg. But these low-fat milk products do not contain any vitamin D.

If you are lactose intolerant, first try lactose-free milk, such as Lactaid and Lacteeze. They are available everywhere. If your gastrointestinal problems persist, soy beverages fortified with 300 mg of calcium per 250 mL (1 cup) and with vitamin D may be an appropriate substitute. They also provide proteins, vitamins and other minerals. Check the label, since many soy beverages are not enriched. If you choose a sparkling drink enriched with calcium, you'll get 300 mg of calcium per 250 mL (1 cup), but no other nutrients.

Unfortunately, it is an error to consider spinach as a good source of calcium. It contains too many oxalates, which impede calcium absorption. Some green leafy vegetables like collards, bok choy, Savoy cabbage and mustard leaves give you less calcium per portion, but the calcium they do contain is easily absorbed, even more so than the calcium in milk. These green vegetables should be part of your daily diet if you want to cut your consumption of milk products without suffering the consequences.

Homemade stock prepared with a chicken carcass that has simmered for several hours with a few spoonfuls of vinegar won't give you the calcium you need. Analyses carried out a few years ago at the University of Arizona showed that such stocks contain very little calcium (8 to 11 mg/250 mL), despite claims to the contrary.

But it's important to remember that calcium is best absorbed when you take it in small doses of 100 to 300 mg at a time in food or as a supplement. You must also take the right dose of vitamin D to make sure the calcium is thoroughly absorbed.

EAT MORE FOODS RICH IN MINERALS LIKE IRON, MAGNESIUM, ZINC, COPPER, MANGANESE AND BORON

Many minerals play an active role in keeping your bones and your blood in balance. They are involved in a number of important reactions, but are unfortunately lacking in many women's diets. As a result, they do not make the contribution they should.

These minerals can be found in many foods. When you consult the tables you will see that some foods are much richer in minerals than others. Legumes, dark green leafy vegetables and whole grains are all good sources of minerals. Foods like liver and oysters are exceptionally rich in iron and zinc.

- You don't have to turn your diet upside down. Just gradually add the best sources of minerals to your menu.
- Sprinkle your cereal with wheat germ or wheat bran, and you get iron, zinc, manganese and magnesium!
- Add legumes to your vegetable soups, salads or casseroles for iron, manganese and magnesium. Try a new recipe based on lentils, chick peas or kidney beans every week.
- Cook leafy green vegetables, spinach or Swiss chard as simply as possible: steamed, or cooked in very little water. Serve with a hint of garlic and olive oil, or incorporate the vegetables into your favourite pasta sauces or into a pizza topping.
- Choose wholegrain breads made from wheat, spelt, rye or multigrains, and make them a permanent part of your diet. Replace white

rice with brown rice. Just these few changes will give you magnesium, fibre, manganese, vitamin B6 and copper. Every mouthful supplies many more nutrients than refined products do.

- Add nuts and avocados to your weekly menu, and you'll easily increase your boron intake.

If you won't eat legumes, green leafy vegetables, whole grains or nuts, it will be very difficult for you to get all the minerals you need.

GET MORE EXERCISE

Physical activity invigorates every part of your body and is a wonderful complement to the suggestions for healthy nutrition you've found in this book. Exercise helps you maintain muscular mass and good bone density, prevents constipation, stimulates the metabolic rate to burn more calories, increases good cholesterol (HDL), lowers blood pressure, reduces insulin resistance and keeps your energy at a high level. Exercise is vital for your well-being; it should be a part of your daily routine.

For a long time, I was a sedentary type and I didn't mind at all. I much preferred reading books and eating broccoli to skiing. Then, in my mid-forties, I changed my life and took up sports and other physical activities. Today, I'm convinced that exercise makes an enormous difference to my quality of life. I can't live without it.

It's never too late to start.

Many researchers have evaluated the impact of exercise on the health of women in general, and of post-menopausal women in particular. They have all recorded positive results. Some conclude that intense, sustained effort is necessary, but others prefer moderate, regular exercise, such as a daily 30-minute walk.

Choose what suits you best. Join a physical fitness club if you like — but it isn't really necessary. You can simply buy a pair of good walking shoes. Be sure to start out gradually and warm up your muscles. Don't rush. Any kind of exercise is good, but ideally, you'll do both aerobic and strength training exercises.

- Use every opportunity you can to make your bones and muscles work.
- Walk as often as you can, and for as long as you can.
- Carry your own parcels.
- Climb the stairs instead of taking the elevator.
- Take up gardening.
- Find a sport you like.
- Become a member of a walking or hiking club.
- Explore your city or town on foot.

Take the appropriate supplement, when necessary

Food is still the best source of the nutrients that are essential to health, but when your normal diet doesn't give you what you need, take a supplement.

Rarely do I meet women who eat sufficient amounts of the important foods. I think supplements can help women benefit from all the essential nutrients if their diet is deficient.

The hormonal changes that come with menopause put additional stress on your entire body, and the risk of deficiency is greater than before menopause. Often, these deficiencies go unnoticed, but they can affect the skin and the bones, as well as the cardiovascular and immune systems. These side effects can be cut to a minimum if you take the right supplement and improve your diet. Choose the supplement that's best for you.

What about multivitamins and minerals? If you have consulted the tables in this book, you have probably realized that your regular diet doesn't contain enough foods rich in minerals other than calcium. You may not be able to meet your needs by relying solely on your diet. In that case, it would be a good idea to take a daily supplement containing adequate amounts of the principal vitamins as well as a whole range of important minerals like manganese, copper, iron, zinc and magnesium. This type of supplement can improve the functioning of the immune system, help calcium do its work, and lower high homocysteine levels (a cardiovascular risk factor). Choose a supplement that provides the following nutrients in dosages not exceeding those indicated.

Doses* of Recommended Nutrients

Vitamin C	80 to 200 mg
Folic acid	400 µg (or 0.4 mg)
Vitamin B6	3 to 5 mg
Iron	10 to 15 mg
Beta-carotene	3,000 to 5,000 IU
Manganese	5 mg
Copper	2.5 mg
Zinc	15 mg

* Higher doses are not recommended.

What about calcium supplements? You don't like milk products or you consume very little or none at all because you're lactose intolerant? You find it difficult to get the calcium you need from other food sources? Then take a calcium supplement to complement what you already get in your food. Tables 28 and 29 on pages 117 and 118 will help you to choose the right supplement and make it a part of your routine.

What about vitamin E supplements? You may have heard that vitamin E can prevent the oxidation of cholesterol and reduce the risk of cardiovascular disease to a minimum, but your diet can supply you with a maximum of only 20 IU a day. A few researchers have observed that taking a vitamin E supplement for more than two years reduced the risk of cardiovascular disease by 40%. Other researchers have noted that taking the supplement can lead to an improvement in immune response. The recommended dose is between 200 and 400 IU a day. Don't exceed this dose, especially if you have high blood pressure or hyperthyroidism or if you take an anticoagulant.

What about evening primrose oil supplements? Evening primrose oil contains gamma-linolenic acid, which the body can utilize more easily than the other two essential fatty acids. This supplement, which has been the subject of a number of studies, does not appear to relieve discomforts specifically related to menopause. It can help ease dry skin problems and premenstrual stress syndrome, however. It can be found in capsule or spray form and is beneficial on the whole.

Still other supplements can complement your diet or help with specific problems. Your dietitian/nutritionist or physician can help you make a wise choice.

The winning formula can taste great!

TABLE 32

Fruits richest* in vitamins, minerals, and dietary fibre

Fruit	Average portion
Guava	1
Watermelon	370 g (2 cups)
Pink or red grapefruit	1/2
Papaya	1/2
Kiwi fruit	2
Cantaloupe	1 quarter
Dried apricots	35 g (1/4 cup)
Orange	1
Strawberries	8
Fresh apricots	4
Blackberries	140 g (1 cup)
Dried peach	40 g (1/4 cup)
Raspberries	130 g (1 cup)
White grapefruit	1/2
Tangerines	1
Persimmons	1
Mangos	1/2
Honeydew melon	1/10
Carambole	1

Source: "Healthy Foods," *Nutrition Action Healthletter*, May 1998.
* Listed in descending order of nutritive value.

TABLE 33
Vegetables richest* in vitamins, minerals, and dietary fibre

Vegetable	Average portion
Collards, cooked	70 g (1/2 cup)
Spinach, cooked	90 g (1/2 cup)
Kale	65 g (1/2 cup)
Swiss chard, cooked	65 g (1/2 cup)
Red pepper	40 g (1/2 pepper)
Sweet potato, cooked without skin	130 g (1 medium)
Pumpkin	120 g (1/2 cup)
Carrots, cooked or raw	80 g (1/2 cup)
Broccoli, cooked	80 g (1/2 cup)
Okra	1/2 cup
Brussels sprouts	82 g (1/2 cup)
Potato, baked in oven with skin	1
Winter squash	125 g (1/2 cup)
Green pepper	40 g (1/2 pepper)
Fresh parsley	16 g (1/4 cup)
Snow peas, cooked	75 g (1/2 cup)
Frozen green peas	85 g (1/2 cup)

Source: *Nutrition Action Healthletter*, 1997.
*Listed in descending order of nutritive value.

Bibliography

Introduction

Campion, E. W. Aging better. *The New England Journal of Medicine*, 1998; 338(15): 1064–1066.

Most women have a positive view of menopause. *North American Menopause Society*, 1997.

Vita, A. J. et al. Aging, health risks, and cumulative disability. *The New England Journal of Medicine*, 338(15): 1035–1041.

Weight

Aloia, J. F. et al. The influence of menopause and hormonal replacement therapy on body cell mass and body fat mass. *American Journal of Obstetrics and Gynecology*, 1995; 172(3): 896–900.

Andersson, B. et al. Influence of menopause on dietary treatment of obesity. *Journal of Internal Medicine*, 1990; 227: 173–181.

Andres, R. et al. Long-term effects of change in body weight on all-cause mortality. A review. *Annals of Internal Medicine*, 1993; 119: 737–743.

Bongain, A. et al. Obesity in obstetrics and gynecology. *European Journal of Obstetrics & Gynecologic Reproductive Biology*, 1998; 77: 217–228

Brzezinski, A. and J. J. Wurtman. Managing weight through the transition years. *Menopause Management*, 1993; 18–23.

Curfman, G. D. Diet Pills Redux. *The New England Journal of Medicine*, 1997; 337(9): 629–630.

Espeland, M. A. et al. Effect of postmenopausal hormone therapy on body weight and waist and hip girths. *Journal of Clinical Endocrinology and Metabolism*, 1997; 82(5): 1549–1556.

Heini, A. F. and R. L. Weinsier. Divergent trends in obesity and fat intake patterns: the American paradox. *The American Journal of Medicine*, 1997; 102: 259–264.

Kahn, H. S. et al. Stable behaviors associated with adults' 10-year change in body mass index and likelihood of gain at the waist. *American Journal of Public Health*, 1997; 87(5): 747–754.

Kassirer, J. P. and M. Angell. Losing weight — an ill fated New Year's resolution. *The New England Journal of Medicine*, 1998; 338(1): 52–54.

Khoo S. K. et al. Hormone Therapy in women in the menopause transition. Randomized, double blind, placebo-controlled trial of effects on body weight, blood pressure, lipo protein levels, anti thrombin III activity and the endometrium. *Medical Journal of Australia*, 1998; 5: 216–220.

Kirchengast, S. et al. Menopause-associated differences in female fat patterning estimated by dual-energy X-ray absorptiometry. *Annals of Human Biology*, 1997; 24(1): 45–54.

Kirtz-Silverstein, D. and E. Barrett-Connor. Long-term post-menopausal hormone use, obesity, and fat distribution in older women. *Journal of American Association*, 1996; 275(1): 46–49.

Langlois, J. A. et al. Weight change between age 50 years and old age is associated with risk of hip fracture in white women aged 67 years and older. *Archives of Internal Medicine*, 1996; 156(9): 989–994.

Lee, I. M. and R. S. Paffenbarger Jr. Is weight loss hazardous? *Nutrition Reviews*, 1996; 54: S116–S124.

Lemieux, S. et al. Seven-year changes in body fat and visceral adipose tissue in women. Association with indexes of plasma glucose-insulin homeostasis. *Diabetes Care*, 1996; 19(9): 983–991.

Melanson, K. J. et al. Fat oxidation in response to four graded energy challenges in younger and older women. *American Journal of Clinical Nutrition*, 1997; 66: 860–866.

Meyer, H. E. et al. Changes in body weight and incidence of hip fracture among middle aged Norwegians. *British Medical Journal*, 1995; 311(6997): 91–92.

Pasquali, R. et al. Body weight, fat distribution and the menopausal status in women. *International Journal of Obesity*, 195; 18: 614–621.

Pouillès, J. M. et al. Influence of body weight variations on the rate of bone loss at the beginning of menopause. *Annales d'Endocrinologie*, 1995; 56(6): 585–589.

Reubinoff, B. E. et al. Effects of hormone replacement therapy on weight, body composition, fat distribution, and food intake in early post-menopausal women: a prospective study. *Fertility and Sterility*, 1995; 64(5): 963–968.

Stevens, J. et al. The effect of age on the association between body-mass index and mortality. *The New England Journal of Medicine*, 1998; 338(1): 1–7.

Taylor, R. W. et al. Body mass index, waist girth, and waist-to-hip ratio as indexes of total and regional adiposity in women: evaluation using receiver operation characteristic curves. *American Journal of Clinical Nutrition*, 1998; 67: 44–49.

Thompson, J. L. et al. Effects of diet and exercise on energy expenditure in postmenopausal women. *American Journal of Clinical Nutrition*, 1997; 66: 867–873.

Turcato, E. et al. Interrelationships between weight loss, body fat distribution and sex hormones in pre- and postmenopausal obese women. *Journal of Internal Medicine*, 1997; 241(5): 363–372.

Wardlaw, G. M. Putting body weight and osteoporosis into perspective. *American Journal of Clinical Nutrition*, 1996; 63(3) Suppl.: 433S–436S.

Wing, R. R. et al. Environmental and familial contributions to insulin levels and change in insulin levels in middle-aged women. *Journal of the American Medical Association*, 1992; 268(14): 1890–1895.

Wurtman, J. Changement dans le poids à la ménopause. *Une véritable amie*, 1992; 9: 9–12.

Hot Flashes

Adlercreutz, C. H. Dietary phyto-oestrogens and the menopause in Japan. *The Lancet*, 1992; 339(8803): 1233.

Adlercreutz, C. H. et al. Urinary excretion of lignans and isoflavonoid phy-toestrogens in Japanese men and women consuming traditional Japanese diet. *American Journal of Clinical Nutrition*, 1991; 54: 1093–1100.

Albertazzi, P. et al. The effect of soy supplementation on hot flushes. *Obstetrics and Gynecology*, 1998; 91(1): 6–10.

Bolton-Smith, C. et al. Evidence for age-related differences in the fatty acid composition of human adipose tissue, independent of diet. *European Journal of Clinical Nutrition*, 1997; 51(9): 619–624.

Brzezinski, A. et al. Short-term effects of phytoestrogens-rich diet on post-menopausal women. *Menopause: The Journal of the North American Menopause Society*, 1997; 4(2): 89–94.

Chenoy, R. et al. Effect of oral gamolenic acid from evening primrose oil on menopausal flushing. *British Medical Journal*, 1994; 308(6927): 501–503.

Dalais, F. S. et al. Effects of dietary phytoestrogens in postmenopausal women. 8th International Congress on the Menopause, Sydney, 1996.

Dwyer, J. T. et al. Tofu and soy drinks contain phytoestrogens. *Journal of the American Dietetic Association*, 1994; 94: 739–743.

Eldridge, A. C. Determination of isoflavones in soybean flours, protein concentrates, and isolates. *Journal of Agriculture and Food Chemistry*, 1982; 30: 353–355.

Hirata, J. D. et al. Does dong quai have estrogenic effects in postmenopausal women? A double-blind, placebo-controlled trial. *Fertility and Sterility*, 1997; 68(6): 981–986.

Horrobin, D. F. Loss of delta-6-desaturase activity as a key factor in aging. *Medical Hypotheses*, 1981; 7(9): 1211–1220.

Knight, D. C. and J. A. Eden. A review of the clinical effects of phytoestrogens. *Obstetrics and Gynecology*, 1996; 87(5): 867–903.

Lock, M. Contested meaning of the menopause. *The Lancet*, 1991; 337: 1270–1272.

Murkies, A. L. et al. Clinical review 92: Phytoestrogens. *Journal of Clinical Endocrinology and Metabolism*, 1998; 83(2): 297–303.

Ordre professionnel des diététistes du Québec. *Analyse de produit: vitamine E.* Comité sur les produits naturels, fiche 002, 1998.

Shaw C. R. The perimenopausal hot flash: epidemiology, physiology and treatment. *Nurse Practice*, 1997; 22(3): 55–56, 61–66.

Wang, H. J. and P. A. Murphy. Isoflavone content in commercial soybean food. *Journal of Agriculture and Food Chemistry*, 1994; 42: 1666–1673.

Arteries

Anderson, J. W. et al. Meta-analysis of the effects of soy protein intake on serum lipids. *The New England Journal of Medicine*, 1995; 333(5): 276–282.

Bouchard, C. *Les maladies cardiovasculaires chez la femme: Formation continue*, Ordre professionnel des diététistes du Québec, 1997.

Byers, T. Hardened fats, hardened arteries? *The New England Journal of Medicine*, 1997; 337(21): 1544–1545.

de Lorgeril, M. et al. Mediterranean diet, traditional risk factors, and the rate of cardiovascular complications after myocardial infarctus. Final report of the Lyon Diet Heart Study. *Circulation*, 1999; 99: 779–785.

de Lorgeril, M. et al. Effect of Mediterranean type of diet on the rate of cardiovascular complications in patients with artery disease. *Journal of the American College of Cardiology*, 1996: 28: 1103–1108.

Garland, M. et al. The relation between dietary intake and adipose tissue composition of selected fatty acids in U.S. women. *American Journal of Clinical Nutrition*, 1998; 67: 25–30.

Gavaler, J. S. et al. An international study of the relationship between alcohol consumption and postmenopausal estradiol levels. *Alcohol and Alcoholism. Supplement*, 1991; 1: 327–330.

Ginsburg, E. S. et al. Effects of alcohol ingestion on estrogens in postmenopausal women. *Journal of the American Medical Association*, 1996; 276: 1747–1751.

Hu, F. B. et al. Dietary intake of alpha linolenic acid and risk of fatal ischemic heart disease among women. *American Journal of Clinical Nutrition*, 1999; 69: 860–867.

Hu, F. B. et al. Dietary intake and the risk of coronary heart disease in women. *The New England Journal of Medicine*, 1997; 337(21): 1491–1499.

Hu, F. B. et al. Frequent nut consumption and risk of coronary heart disease in women: prospective cohort study. *British Medical Journal*, 1998; 317: 1341–1345.

Hulley, S. et al. Randomized trial of oestrogen plus progestin for secondary prevention of coronary heart disease in postmenopausal women. *Journal of the American Medical Association*, 1998; 280: 605–613.

JAMA and The Archives Journals editors. Estrogen replacement therapy and heart disease: a discussion of the PEPI trial. *Archives Journal Club/Women's Health*, WEB, 1997.

Jeppesen, J. et al. Effects of low-fat, high-carbohydrate diets on risk factors for ischemic heart disease in postmenopausal women. *American Journal of Clinical Nutrition*, 1997; 65: 1027–1033.

Kjekshus, J. and T. R. Pedersen. Reducing the risk of coronary events: evidence from the Scandinavian Simvastatin Survival Study (4S). *The American Journal of Cardiology*, 1995; 64C–68C.

Lapidus, L. et al. Dietary habits in relation to incidence of cardiovascular disease and death in women: a 12 year follow-up of participants in the population study of women in Gothenburg, Sweden. *American Journal of Clinical Nutrition*, 1986; 44: 444–448.

Nestel, P. J. et al. Soy isoflavones improve systemic arterial compliance but not plasma lipids in menopausal and perimenopausal women. *Arteriosclerosis Thrombosis Vascular Biology*, 1997; 17(12): 3392–3398.

Newnham, H. H. and J. Silberberg. Women's hearts are hard to break. *The Lancet*, 1997; 349 (suppl. I): sI3–sI6.

Petitti, D. B. Hormone replacement therapy and heart disease prevention. Experimentation trumps observation. *Journal of the American Medical Association*, 1998; 280: 650–652.

Poehlman, E. T. et al. Menopause-associated changes in plasma lipids, insulin-like growth factor I and blood pressure: a longitudinal study. *European Journal of Clinical Investigations*, 1997; 27(4): 322–326.

Portaluppi, F. et al. Relative influence of menopausal status, age, and body mass index on blood pressure. *Hypertension*, 1997; 29(4): 976–979.

Renaud, S. et al. Cretan Mediterranean diet for prevention of coronary heart disease. *American Journal of Clinical Nutrition*, 1995; 61 (suppl.): 1360S–1367S.

Ridker, P. M. et al. Homocysteine and risk of cardiovascular disease among postmenopausal women. *Journal of the American Medical Association*, 1999; 281: 1817–1821.

Shelley, J. M. et al. Relationship of endogenous sex hormones to lipids and blood pressure in mid-aged women. *Annals of Epidemiology*, 1998; 8(1): 39–45.

Simkin-Silverman, L. et al. Prevention of cardiovascular risk factor elevations in healthy premenopausal women. *Prevention Medicine*, 1995; 24(5): 509–517.

Sitruk-Ware, R. Cardiovascular risk at the menopause — Role of sexual steroids. *Hormonal Resource*, 1995; 43: 58–63.

Stefanick, M. L. et al. Effects of diet and exercise in men and postmenopausal women with low levels of HDL cholesterol and high levels of LDL cholesterol. *The New England Journal of Medicine*, 1998; 339(1): 12–20.

Sundram, K. et al. Trans (elaidic) fatty acids adversely affect the lipoprotein profile relative to specific saturated fatty acids in humans. *Journal of Nutrition*, 1997; 127(3): 514S–520S.

Thomas, J. L. et al. Coronary artery disease in women. *Archives of Internal Medicine*, 1998; 158: 333–337.

Tikkanen, M. J. et al. Effect of soybean phytoestrogen intake on low density lipoprotein oxidation resistance. *Proceedings National Academy of Sciences USA*, 1998; 95(6): 3106–3110.

Tinker, L. F. Diabetes mellitus — a priority health care issue for women. *Journal of the American Dietetic Association*, 1994; 94(9): 976–985.

van Beresteijn Emerentia, C. H. et al. Perimenopausal increase in serum cholesterol: A 10 year longitudinal study. *American Journal of Epidemiology*, 1993; 137(4): 383–392.

Willeit, J. et al. The role of insulin in age-related sex differences of cardio-vascular risk profile and morbidity. *Atherosclerosis*, 1997; 130(1-2): 183–189.

Williams, M. J. et al. Regional fat distribution in women and risk of cardio-vascular disease. *American Journal of Clinical Nutrition*, 1997; 65: 855–860.

Osteoporosis

Albala, C. et al. Obesity as a protective factor for postmenopausal osteoporo-sis. *International Journal of Obesity & Related Metabolic Disorders*, 1996; 20(11): 1027–1032.

Atkinson, S. Avoiding the fracture zone. Calcium: why get more? *Nutrition Action Healthletter*, 1998; 25(3): 3–7.

Barzel, U. S. Dietary patterns and blood pressure. *The New England Journal of Medicine*, 1997; 337(9): 636.

Chiu, J. F. et al. Long-term vegetarian diet and bone mineral density in post-menopausal Taiwanese women. *Calcified Tissue International*, 1997; 60: 245–249.

Curchan, G. C. et al. Comparison of dietary calcium with supplemental cal-cium and other nutrients as factors affecting the risk for kidney stones in women. *Annals of Internal Medicine*, 1997; 126: 497–504.

Dawson-Hughes, B. Osteoporosis treatment and the calcuim requirement. *American Journal of Clinical Nutrition*, 1998; 67: 5–6.

Dawson-Hughes, B. et al. Effect of calcium and vitamin D supplementation on bone density in men and women 65 years of age or older. *The New England Journal of Medicine*, 1997; 337(10): 670–676.

Franceschi, S. et al. The influence of body size, smoking, and diet on bone density in pre- and postmenopausal women. *Epidemiology*, 1996; 7(4): 411–414.

Heaney, R. P. Bone mass, nutrition, and other lifestyle factors. *Nutrition Reviews*, 1996; 54(4): S3–S10.

Hosking, D. et al. Prevention of bone loss with alendronate in post-menopausal women under 60 years of age. *The New England Journal of Medicine*, 1998; 338(8): 485–492.

Institute of Medicine, Food and Nutrition Board. National Academy of Sciences. *Dietary References intake for calcium, phosphorus, magnesium, vita-min D and fluoride*, National Academy Press, Washington D.C., 1997.

Itoh, R. et al. Dietary protein intake and urinary excretion of calcium: a cross-sectional study in a healthy Japanese population. *American Journal of Clinical Nutrition*, 1998; 67: 438–444.

Jamal, S. A. et al. Warfarin use and risk for osteoporosis in elderly women. *Annals of Internal Medicine*, 1998; 128: 829–832.

Kanis, J. A. et al. The diagnosis of osteoporosis. *Journal of Bone and Mineral Research*, 1994; 9(8): 1137–1141.

Kaufman, J. M. Role of calcium and vitamin D in the prevention and the treatment of postmenopausal osteoporosis: an overview. *Clinical Rheumatology*, 1995; 14(3) Suppl.: 9–13.

Meacham, S. L. Effect of boron supplementation on blood and urinary calcium, magnesium, and phosphorus, and urinary boron in athletic and sedentary women. *American Journal of Clinical Nutrition*, 1995; 61(2): 341–345.

Michelson, D. et al. Bone mineral density in women with depression. *The New England Journal of Medicine*, 1996; 335: 1176–1181.

Naghii, M. R. et al. The boron content of selected foods and the estimation of its daily intake among free-living subjects. *Journal of the American College of Nutrition*, 1996; 15(6): 614–619.

Newnham, R. E. Essentiality of boron for healthy bones and joints. *Environmental Health Perspectives*, 1994; 102 (suppl. 7): 83–85.

Nielsen, F. H. Biochemical and physiologic consequences of boron deprivation in humans. *Environmental Health Perspectives*, 1994; 102(suppl. 7): 59–63.

Nieves, J. W. et al. Calcium potentiates the effect of estrogen and calcitonin on bone mass: review and analysis. *American Journal of Clinical Nutrition*, 1998; 67: 18–24.

Prince, R. L. Diet and the prevention of osteoporotic fractures. *The New England Journal of Medicine*, 1997; 337(10): 701.

Reid, I. R. Therapy of osteoporosis: calcium vitamin D, and exercise. *American Journal of Medical Science*, 1996; 312(6): 278–286.

Reid, I. R. et al. Long-term effects of calcium supplementation on bone loss and fractures in postmenopausal women: a randomized controlled trial. *American Journal of Medicine*, 1995; 98(4): 331–335.

Strause, L. et al. Spinal bone loss in postmenopausal women supplemented with calcium and trace minerals. *Journal of Nutrition*, 1994; 124(7): 1060–1064.

Suleiman, S. et al. Effect of calcium intake and physical activity level on bone mass and turnover in healthy, white, postmenopausal women. *American Journal of Clinical Nutrition*, 1997; 66: 937–943.

Tucker, K. L. et al. Potassium, magnesium, and fruit and vegetable intakes are associated with greater bone mineral density in elderly men and women. *American Journal of Clinical Nutrition*, 1999; 69: 727–736.

Utiger, R. D. The need for more vitamin D. *The New England Journal of Medicine*, 1998; 338(12): 828.

Van Loan, M. D. et al. Effect of weight loss on bone mineral content and bone mineral density in obese women. *American Journal of Clinical Nutrition*, 1998; 67: 734–738.

Volpe, S. L. et al. The relationship between boron and magnesium status and bone mineral density in the human: a review. *Magnesium Research*, 1993; 6(3): 291–296.

Cancer

Adlercreutz, C. H. et al. Dietary phytoestrogens and cancer: *in vitro* and *in vivo* studies. *Journal of Steroid Biochemistry & Molecular Biology*, 1992; 41(308): 331–337.

Adlercreutz, C. H. et al. Soybean phytoestrogens intake and cancer risk. *Journal of Nutrition*, 1995; 125 (3 Suppl.): 757S–770S.

Adlercreutz, C. H. and W. Mazur. Phyto-oestrogens and Western diseases. *Annals of Medicine*, 1997; 29(2): 95–120.

Berrino, F. et al. A randomized trial to prevent hormonal patterns at high risk for breast cancer: the DIANA (diet and androgens) project. Milan, Italy: Instituto Nazional Tumori, 1997.

Bordonada, R. et al. Alcohol intake and risk of breast cancer: the Euramic study. *Neoplasma*, 1997; 44(3): 150–156.

Cohen, L. A. et al. A rationale for dietary intervention in postmenopausal breast cancer patients: an update. *Nutrition and Cancer*, 1993; 19(1): 1–10.

Freudenheim, J. L. et al. Premenopausal breast cancer risk and intake of vegetables, fruits, and related nutrients. *Journal of the National Cancer Institute*, 1996; 88(6): 340–348.

Goodman, M. T. et al. Association of soy and fiber consumption with the risk of endometrial cancer. *American Journal of Epidemiology*, 1997; 146: 294–306.

Horn-Ross, P. L. Phytoestrogens, body composition, and breast cancer. *Cancer Causes Control*, 1995; 6(6): 567–573.

Ingram, D. et al. Case control study of phyto-oestrogens and breast cancer (see comments). *The Lancet*, 1997; 350: 990–994.

Longnecker, M. P. et al. Intake of carrots, spinach, and supplements containing vitamin A in relation to risk of breast cancer. *Cancer Epidemiology, Biomarkers and Prevention*, 1997; 6(11): 887–892.

Martin, M. E. et al. Interactions between phytoestrogens and human sex steroid binding protein. *Life Science*, 1996; 58(5): 429–436.

Messina, M. J. et al. Soy intake and cancer risk: a review of the *in vitro* and *in vivo* data. *Nutrition and Cancer*, 1994; 21(2): 113–131.

Schardt, D. Phytochemicals: plants against cancer. *Nutrition Action Healthletter*, 1994; 21(3): 9–11.

Smith-Warner, S. A. et al. Alcohol and breast cancer in women: A pooled analysis of cohort studies. *Journal of the American Medical Association*, 1998; 279(7): 535–540.

Steinmetz, K. A. and J. D. Potter. Vegetables, fruit, and cancer prevention. A review. *Journal of the American Dietetic Association*, 1996; 96: 1027–1039.

Stoll, B. A. Eating to beat breast cancer: potential role for soy supplement. *Annals of Oncology*, 1997; 8(3): 223–225.

Thune, I. et al. Physical activity and the risk of breast cancer. *The New England Journal of Medicine*, 1997; 336(18): 1269–1275.

Winston, J. C. Phytochemicals: guardians of our health. *Journal of the American Dietetic Association*, 1996; 5(3): 6–8.

Yan, L. et al. Dietary flaxseed supplementation and experimental metastasis of melanoma cells in mice. *Cancer Letter*, 1998; 124(2): 181–186.

Zava, D. T. and G. Duwe. Estrogenic and antiproliferative properties of genistein and other flavonoids in human breast cancer cells *in vitro*. *Nutrition and Cancer*, 1997; 27(1): 31–40.

Zhang, S. et al. Better breast cancer survival for postmenopausal women who are less overweight and eat less fat. The Iowa Women's Health Study. *Cancer*, 1995; 76(2): 275–283.

Zumoff, B. Does postmenopausal estrogen administration increase the risk of breast cancer? Contributions of animal, biochemical, and clinical investigative studies to a resolution of the controversy. *Proceedings of Society for Experimental Biology and Medicine*, 1998; 217(1): 30–37.

The Winning Formula for Menopause

Appel, L. J. et al. A clinical trial of the effects of dietary patterns on blood pressure. *The New England Journal of Medicine*, 1997; 336(16): 1117–1124.

Chandra, R. J. Effect of vitamin and trace-element supplementation on immune responses and infection in elderly subjects. *The Lancet*, 1992; 340: 1124–1127.

Chandra, R. J. Graying of the immune system; can nutrient supplements improve immunity in the elderly? *Journal of the American Medical Association*, 1997; 227(17): 1398–1399.

Choay, P. et al. Value of micronutriment supplements in the prevention or correction of disorders accompanying menopause. *Revue française de gynécologie et obstétrique*, 1990; 85(12): 702–705.

Connell Hadfield, L. et al. Calcium content of soup stocks with added vinegar. *Journal of the American Dietetic Association*, 1989; 89: 1810–1811.

Houde Nadeau, M. La biodisponibilité de calcium. *Diététique en action*, 1998; 12(1): 11–13.

Kushi, L. H. et al. Dietary antioxidant vitamins and death from coronary heart disease in postmenopausal women. *The New England Journal of Medicine*, 1996; 334(18): 1156–1162.

Oakley, G. P. Eat right and take a multivitamin. *The New England Journal of Medicine*, 1998; 338(15): 1060–1061.

Rimm, E. B. Folate and vitamin B6 from diet and supplements in relation to risk of coronary heart disease among women. *Journal of the American Medical Association*, 1998; 279: 359–364.

Stampfer, M. J. et al. Vitamin E consumption and the risk of coronary disease in women. *The New England Journal of Medicine*, 1993; 328(20): 1444–1449.

Nutritional Values of Foods

Brault-Dubuc, M. and Caron Lahaie. *Valeur nutritive des aliments*, Société Brault-Lahaie, Saint-Lambert, 1994.

Hands, E. S. *Food Finder, food sources of vitamins and minerals*, ESHA Research, United States, 1990.

Recommended Nutrient Intakes

Health and Welfare Canda. *Nutrition recommendations*, Report of the Scientific Review Committee, 1990.

Adequate Intakes

Institute of Medicine, Food and Nutrition Board. National Academy of Sciences. *Dietary References intake for calcium, phosphorus, magnesium, vitamin D and fluoride*, National Academy Press, Washington D.C., 1997.

Soy Recipes

Jarobi, D. *SOY!*, Rocklin, CA, Prima Publications, 1996.

Melina, V. and J. Forest. *Cooking Vegetarian*, Toronto, Macmillan, 1996.

Mitchell, P. *The Complete Soy Cookbook*, New York, Macmillan, 1998.

Paino, J., and L. Messinger. *The Tofu Book*, New York, Avery Publishing Group, 1991.

Sass, L. *The New Soy Cookbook*, San Francisco, Chronicle Books, 1998.

Index

dangers of excess, 22, 123
distribution, 10
intra-abdominal, 10,
11–12, 22
fatigue, menopausal, 3
causes of, 26–31, 66
dietary solutions for,
31–34, 132
and eating habits, 27–34
and exercise, 138
and insulin levels, 28,
30–31
and iron deficiency,
29–30
and thyroid gland, 30
fats, 75–77. *See also* oils
and breast cancer, 122,
127
and calcium absorption,
85
and cardiovascular
disease, 6, 75–77, 135
and cholesterol, 75–77
consumption of, 20, 75–77
effects on body of, 50
good, 19, 76–77, 129, 135
health risks of, 73
in healthy diet, 129, 135
hydrogenated (bad), 6,
19, 50, 72, 77, 122, 127
monounsaturated (good),
76, 135
omega-3 (good), 76, 122,
123, 127, 133, 135
saturated (bad), 6, 28, 50,
76, 122, 127
fenfluramine, 6
ferritin, 30, 34. *See also* iron
fibre, dietary
and bone density, 85
and breast cancer, 123–24
and cholesterol, 78
and constipation, 7, 63
in healthy diet, 64
insoluble, 78
soluble, 78
sources of, 64, 67 (table)
fibrinogen, 79
fish
as part of healthy diet,
18, 33, 131

as source of omega-3
fats, 76, 123
flavonoids, 125. *See also*
fruits
flaxseed
and breast cancer, 123,
125–26
in healthy diet, 18, 46,
129, 133
and hot flashes, 44–45
as omega-3 fat source,
76, 135
as phytoestrogen source,
43, 44, 46, 123, 125
flaxseed oil, 125
folic acid. *See also* vitamin
B-complex
deficiency of, 7, 74–75
recommended amounts
of, 140
sources of, 82–83 (table)
as supplement, 78–79,
140
Fosamax, 112
fruits
and bone density, 85, 90
and breast cancer, 125,
127
as fibre source, 78, 142
(table)
in healthy diet, 18, 19–20,
49, 129, 132, 133–35
and hot flashes, 45, 49
insufficient intake of, 7
and iron absorption, 29,
34
as nutrient source, 78,
142 (table)

gamma-linolenic acid, 50,
141
glands
adrenal, 14, 123
pancreas, 30
thyroid, 7, 30, 31, 79, 141
grains. *See* whole grains

HDL. *See* cholesterol, good
Heart and Estrogen/Pro-
gestin Replacement
Study (HERS), 71

heart disease. *See* cardiovascular disease
heel ultrasound, 110–11
hemoglobin, 30, 34. *See also*
iron
high blood pressure
and cardiovascular
disease, 70, 71, 73
and diet, 133
and exercise, 138
and vitamin E, 79, 141
homocysteine
lowering, 140
test for levels of, 75
and vitamin B, 74–75,
78–79
hormone replacement
therapy, xi
and bone loss, 112
and calcium supplements,
15–16, 113
and cardiovascular
disease, 71–72
compared to phyto-
estrogens, 44, 78
and iron deficiency,
29–30
research studies on,
15–16, 22, 71–72, 79
and smoking, 16, 22
and weight gain, 16–17
and wine-drinking, 79
hormones. *See also* names of
specific hormones
and breast cancer, 122–25
and cardiovascular
disease, 70–72
and prostoglandins, 50
sex, 14, 124, 127
and weight gain, 15–16
hot flashes, 3, 26, 42–61
and diet, 45–50
in Japanese women,
42–43
and phytoestrogens,
43–45, 46, 50, 133
research studies on,
44–45, 50
hydrogenated fats, 6, 19,
50, 72, 77, 122, 127.
See also trans fatty acids